BASIC PHYSICS IN RADIOLOGY

BASIC PHYSICS IN RADIOLOGY

L. A. W. KEMP

B.Sc,. Ph.d., F.INST.P.

Formerly Chief Physicist to the London Hospital
Senior Principal Scientific Officer
Division of Radiation Science
National Physical Laboratory,
Teddington, Middlesex

AND

R. OLIVER

M.A., D.Sc., F.INST.P., F.I.E.E., M.I.BIOL.

Chief Physicist in the Department of
Radiation Physics of the United Oxford Hospitals
Radiation Protection Officer
University of Oxford

SECOND EDITION

Blackwell Scientific Publications
Oxford and Edinburgh

FIRST PUBLISHED 1959
SECOND EDITION 1970

Printed in Great Britain by
WESTERN PRINTING SERVICES LTD, BRISTOL
and bound by
THE KEMP HALL BINDERY

CONTENTS

24360

PREFACE
TO SECOND EDITION

This volume, like its predecessor, attempts to provide a concise treatment of the basic physical principles relevant to the study of radiology. It is not a 'cram' book, but includes, wherever possible, examples and exercises closely related to this subject. It is intended as a companion volume to 'Mathematics for Radiographers'* and to 'Radiation Physics in Radiology',† but should be a useful introduction to physics in conjunction with any of the more specialized radiological texts. The general arrangement of the First Edition has been retained, so as to minimize confusion where both books are in use in the same class. However, in the interests of economy, some matter, less related to a radiological syllabus, has had to be dropped and this has necessitated some rearrangement of the remainder.

The question of units has also had to be reconsidered. The metric system of units is now universal in scientific work and increasingly in everyday use. Therefore, the traditional British units (the pound and foot) have only been retained in the general treatment of the initial chapters. The so-called S.I. units (involving the kilogramme, metre, newton and joule) are now recommended, and these (in particular the newton as a unit of force) have been introduced. However, as the older Metric (C.G.S.) units will still be found by the student in many other books, these (involving the gramme, centimetre, dyne and erg) have been retained and used where appropriate.

The mathematical proofs (previously Appendix III) have been dropped, as these can be found in other physics books if the student is particularly interested. Biographical notes (Appendix IV) have been regarded as expendable and Examination Questions (Appendix V) have been left out as these 'date' quickly with the changing emphasis in the papers set.

* 'Mathematics for Radiographers', L. A. W. Kemp, Blackwell Scientific Publications, Oxford, 1964.

† 'Radiation Physics in Radiology', R. Oliver, Blackwell Scientific Publications, Oxford, 1966.

CHAPTER 1

Introductory Notes on the Structure and Properties of Matter

ATOMS AND MOLECULES; ELEMENTS AND COMPOUNDS

The idea that matter is composed of tiny particles called *atoms*, too small to be seen individually, is by no means new. It emerged in ancient Greek thought, and the *atomic theory*, as it may be called, can be traced among the theories of subsequent philosophers, right up to the nineteenth century and the time of the Englishman John Dalton, whose own particular version of it (put forward in 1810) laid the foundations of modern chemistry.

Briefly stated, Dalton's atomic theory suggested that *all* matter, whether solid, liquid or gas, was composed of these tiny particles called atoms, and that all the atoms of a given *element* (which Robert Boyle over a hundred years before had defined as a substance which could not be split into any other—simpler—substances) had the same size and weight, and differed from the atoms of all other elements. These atoms, Dalton suggested, were capable of combining with one or more atoms either of the same element or of another element to form *molecules*.

Molecules, each containing the same combination of atoms of different elements, form the basis of the class of substances known as *compounds*. Thus the gas *hydrogen* and the gas *chlorine* are both elements, but when they combine together each hydrogen atom pairs off with an atom of chlorine, and molecules of the compound hydrogen chloride are formed. This combining together can occur even among atoms of the same element. For example, ordinary gaseous oxygen consists of oxygen *molecules* each containing two oxygen atoms.

SOLIDS, LIQUIDS AND GASES

In *solids* the atoms (or molecules, as the case may be) occupy fixed positions relative to each other, and only by the application of comparatively large forces can their relative positions be changed. Nevertheless the atoms are vibrating rapidly about their mean positions. The application of heat causes this vibration to increase (the temperature rises), and when the vibration becomes sufficiently violent the atoms (or molecules) break away from their fixed positions, and begin to move about among each other: the *liquid* state has been reached. If the liquid is heated sufficiently, the speed of the particles becomes so great that they escape in large numbers through the surface of the liquid, to become a *gas*. In the gaseous state the molecules (or atoms) are much further apart than in the liquid state, and spread out as freely-moving particles to fill the whole of the available space.

THE KINETIC THEORY OF GASES

It is seen that a gas under ordinary conditions is composed of atoms or molecules moving rapidly in a random manner amongst each other, and separated on an average by distances large compared with the size of the particles. This concept of a gas forms the basis of the so-called *kinetic theory* of gases. According to this theory, there will be continual collisions of the particles with the walls of the vessel containing the gas. This bombardment is responsible for the phenomenon which we call the *pressure* of the gas. It may now be seen why increasing the temperature (or decreasing the volume) of a given quantity of gas increases its pressure: for an increase of temperature brings about an increase in the speed at which the particles strike the walls of the containing vessel, whilst a decrease in volume will obviously decrease the average distance between the particles, and therefore increase the *number* of them which strike a given area of the walls in a given time. In either case the intensity of bombardment of the walls of the containing vessel is increased, and the pressure rises.

The Pressure of the Atmosphere

The atmosphere consists of a mixture of gases, the chief of which are nitrogen and oxygen. There are also traces of other gases present, and, except in unusual circumstances, water vapour as well. Each constituent of the atmosphere will exert a pressure, the sum total of which is called the pressure of the atmosphere.

This pressure is usually measured by finding the height of the column of mercury which it is capable of supporting. One reason why mercury is chosen for this purpose is that as it is a very heavy liquid the height of it which the atmosphere can support is not inconveniently large (if water were used the height would be some 30 feet!). The mercury is incorporated in an instrument called a *barometer*. A simple form of this instrument consists of a U-tube of glass, one side of which is much taller than the other, and is sealed off at the top. The shorter arm is open to the atmosphere. Mercury is poured into the open end of the tube, which is held in such a manner that the mercury fills the whole of the longer arm and part of the shorter arm. The instrument is then arranged with the arms vertical. Mercury runs down the closed arm, thereby raising the level in the open arm, until atmospheric pressure, acting on the surface of the mercury in the latter, is capable of preventing any further movement (Fig. 1a). Practically speaking, an almost perfect vacuum is left above the mercury in the closed arm. The height *h* cm of the mercury in the closed arm remaining above the level of the mercury in the open arm is thus virtually a measure of atmospheric pressure, and is commonly referred to as the *height of the barometer*. An accurate form of this instrument, shown in Fig. 1b, is known as the

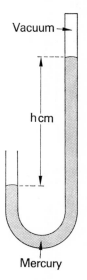

Fig. 1a.
A simple mercury
barometer.

Fortin barometer. At sea level the height of the mercury column supported by the atmosphere is, on the average, about 76 cm, and this value is used as the *standard* (or *normal*) pressure for the purposes of calculation. As it is a measure of the pressure due to the whole atmosphere above the point, the height of the mercury column will obviously decrease with increasing altitude (about 0·9 cm for each 100 m above sea level), and also, of course, the pressure will vary over a range of several centimetres with weather conditions.

THE RELATIONSHIP BETWEEN PRESSURE AND VOLUME OF A GAS— BOYLE'S LAW

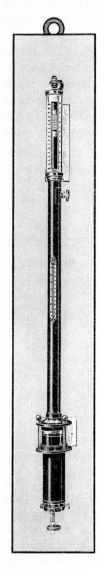

Robert Boyle studied the effect which changing the pressure of a given quantity of gas had on its volume.

He discovered that as the pressure was increased the volume decreased in such a way that doubling one halved the other, trebling one reduced the other to one third of its original value, and so on. Two quantities related in this way are said to be *inversely proportional* to one another.* This law may therefore be stated as follows: '*the volume of a given mass of gas is inversely proportional to its pressure, the temperature remaining constant.*'

It is important to realize that Boyle's Law also allows us to calculate changes in the *mass* of gas contained in the same *volume* at different pressures, a type of calculation necessary in correcting the reading of an X-ray exposure meter for changes in atmospheric pressure. Thus if a mass of gas m_1 gm is contained in a volume V_1 cc at a pressure P_1 cm of mercury, then from Boyle's Law, at a pressure P_2 this same mass of gas will be contained in a volume V_2,

$$\text{where} \qquad \frac{V_2}{V_1} = \frac{P_1}{P_2},$$

$$\text{whence} \qquad V_2 = \frac{P_1}{P_2} \cdot V_1.$$

At this pressure P_2, therefore, a mass of gas m_1 occupies a volume V_2, and the original volume V_1 will now contain a mass of gas m_2,

$$\text{where} \qquad m_2 = \frac{V_1}{V_2} \cdot m_1,$$

Fig. 1b.
A Fortin barometer.

(Photograph by courtesy of Messrs. F. Darton & Co, Ltd, Watford, Herts.)

* See 'Mathematics for Radiographers'' p. 37.

whence, substituting for V_2, $m_2 = \dfrac{V_1}{\left(\dfrac{P_1}{P_2} V_1\right)} \cdot m_1$

$$= \frac{P_2}{P_1} \cdot m_1 ,$$

i.e. $\dfrac{m_2}{m_1} = \dfrac{P_2}{P_1} .$

In words, *the mass of gas contained in a given volume is proportional to its pressure, providing the temperature remains constant.*

It should be noted that the corresponding correction of an exposure meter reading for changes in *temperature* is calculated in a somewhat similar manner by the application of Charles' Law (see p. 61).

EXERCISES

1. State briefly what you know about (a) atoms, (b) molecules.
2. Show how some of the physical differences between solids, liquids, and gases may be described in terms of the Atomic Theory of the structure of matter.
3. What is meant by the *pressure* of a gas? To what may it be attributed?
4. Describe an instrument by means of which the pressure of the atmosphere is measured. What units are usually employed to represent atmospheric pressure?
5. Explain the meaning of inverse proportion.
   State Boyle's Law.
   A certain mass of gas has a volume of 200 cc at normal atmospheric pressure (76 cm of mercury). What would its volume become if the pressure were increased to 95 cm of mercury?
   What is the ratio of the mass of 200 cc of the gas at these two pressures?

CHAPTER 2

Statics—The Study of Forces

SCALARS AND VECTORS

In everyday life we deal with many things of which the size or *magnitude* is the only important feature. This is true, for instance, of sums of money, and quantities of matter measured by mass or volume. These quantities, which we know all about when we have been told their magnitudes, are called *scalars*.

There are many instances, however, when our information is incomplete if we have merely been told the magnitude of something. For instance, it may be stated that an object has been moved 20 ft from its initial position, but we should not know all about the movement—or *displacement* as we shall call it—unless, in addition, we were told its *direction*. Many conventions might be adopted, but for displacements in a horizontal plane the compass directions are useful, and the displacement might be said to be one of 20 ft in, say, a NE direction. A quantity which is not fully defined until we have stated not only its magnitutude (20 ft in the case of the displacement referred to above), but also its direction, is called a *vector*.

Thus scalars have magnitude only, whilst vectors have direction as well as magnitude.

Velocities and Forces as Vectors

Velocity, which is concerned with the *rate* of movement or displacement, is a vector, for we need to state not only the rate, but also the direction if we are to describe it completely.

It is easy to appreciate that a force is also a vector, although it must first be made more clear what exactly we mean by a 'force'. Vaguely it might be defined as a push or pull, but we can be a little more specific if we realize that a push or a pull is usually exerted in order either to set something in motion or to change the speed or direction of something already moving. In fact a *force* may be *defined* as *that which causes stationary objects to move or moving objects to change their speed or direction*. From all this it is clear that the direction in which a force is exerted is as important as its magnitude. Thus forces, too, are vectors.

Units of Force

We are all familiar with the force of gravity: we experience it every time we lift something. In fact by the 'heaviness' or 'weight' of an object is meant simply the magnitude of the force of gravity on it. The bigger this force, the greater the *weight* of the object is said to be. The standard quantity of matter, formerly in Britain the *pound*, is usually to be seen in the form of a special piece of brass or iron used by shopkeepers, in conjunction with 'scales', for 'weighing' purposes. If we pick up a 'pound' we feel the force of gravity on it: we experience the *weight* of one pound, or in short, 1 *pound weight*. The force of gravity on a pound can be used as a unit of force, and we may talk of a force of, say, 10 *pounds weight* (10 lb wt) meaning a force 10 times bigger than the force which gravity exerts on one pound. Similarly, in the Metric system, we may talk of a force of, say, 5 *grammes weight* (5 gm wt), meaning a force 5 times greater than the force which gravity exerts on one gramme. A force of 1 lb wt is about 454 times bigger than a force of 1 gm wt.

The *pound weight* and the *gramme weight* are called the *gravitational* units of force, since they involve the force of gravity.*

Representation of Vectors by Straight Lines

As already seen, to describe vectors fully two pieces of information are necessary, one being a number indicating the *magnitude* of the vector, and the other a statement concerning its *direction*. These two pieces of information may conveniently be combined by representing the vector by a straight line, whose direction represents the direction of the vector, and whose length, to some convenient scale, represents the magnitude of the vector. For instance, suppose it is wished to

---

* It is to be noted that these units are not strictly constant, since the force of gravity on a given object varies slightly at different points on the earth's surface. For our present purpose this variation may be neglected. In Chapter 3 the so-called 'absolute' units of force will be considered, which are independent of gravity, and therefore invariant.

represent in this manner a velocity of 3 mph in a SE direction. The line *AB* (Fig. 2) is drawn 3 units long (each unit representing 1 mph) in a direction bisecting the lines representing the E and S directions. This line *AB* indicates all the necessary information regarding the velocity. Similarly, a force of 2 lb wt acting in a SW direction may be represented by *AC*, as also shown in Fig. 2.

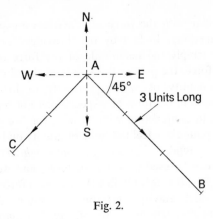

Fig. 2.

EXERCISES

1. Explain the difference between scalars and vectors.
2. Represent each of the following vectors by a straight line drawn to a convenient scale: (a) a displacement of 10 ft in a SW direction, (b) a displacement of 7 metres in a direction due N, (c) a velocity of 15 mph in a direction due E, (d) a velocity of 27 cm per sec in a SE direction, (e) a force of 9 lb wt acting in a direction due W, (f) a force of 3 gm wt acting in a NW direction.

THE PARALLELOGRAM OF FORCES

The total of two scalars (e.g. two sums of money) is obtained simply by adding arithmetically the two numbers representing their magnitudes. Thus £25 and £13 make £38, and so on. The question then arises as to how two *vectors* may be added to find their total or *resultant*.

Suppose a body is acted on simultaneously by two forces at an angle to each other. For example, a trolley may be pulled along by two people exerting forces in the directions shown in plan in Fig. 3, and it is required to find the resultant force on the trolley. There are really two questions here: what is the *magnitude* of the resultant force, and what is its *direction*? Suppose the two forces are 25 lb wt and 13 lb wt respectively. Then the magnitude of the resultant will *not*, in general, be equal to (25 + 13), that is 38 lb wt. In one case only will this be true: when

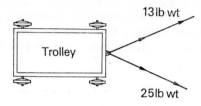

Fig. 3.

the two forces act along the same line, i.e. when the two people in the above example pull together in precisely the same direction. Thus it is seen that, with this exception, vectors cannot be added together in the same way as scalars.

We can discover how they may be added by first considering displacements instead of forces. What is found to be true of displacements will be true of forces and velocities, for they also are vectors. Suppose an X-ray tube at T (Fig. 4) is moved first to X and then to Z, i.e. it is

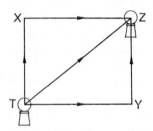

Fig. 4. Movement of the X-ray tube head from T to X and then to Z, or from T to Y and then to Z is equivalent to a single displacement from T to Z as shown.

given two displacements in succession, represented by TX and XZ. Imagine now the impression which would be gained by someone who, after seeing the tube at T, does not see it again until it has reached Z. Such a person would assume that the tube had been moved *direct* from T to Z, i.e. it would seem to have been subject to a single displacement represented by TZ. Thus:

Displacement TX + Displacement XZ = Displacement TZ.

2

Of course the tube could equally well have first been moved to *Y* and then raised to *Z*, i.e. given two displacements represented by *TY* and *YZ*, which again would have been equivalent to the single displacement *TZ*.

In this example the two component displacements are in directions at right angles to one another. Obviously the same argument would apply whatever the angle between them. Thus in Fig. 5, for component

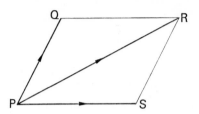

Fig. 5. For component displacements *PQ* and *PS* the resultant displacement is *PR*, the diagonal of the parallelogram formed on *PQ* and *PS* as adjacent sides.

displacements *PQ* and *PS* the resultant displacement is *PR*, the diagonal of the parallelogram formed on *PQ* and *PS* as adjacent sides.

In a similar manner we may say that for two component *forces* acting on an object at *P*, and represented in magnitude and direction by *PQ* and *PS*, the *resultant* force on the object at *P* is represented (again in both magnitude and direction) by the diagonal *PR*. This construction (that of representing the two given forces by the adjacent sides of a parallelogram, and drawing in the diagonal between them to obtain the resultant force) is known as *The Parallelogram of Forces*.

We can now return to the trolley (Fig. 3) pulled along by two people. The two forces produced on the trolley are to be taken as 25 lb wt and 13 lb wt, and in addition let us suppose that the angle between the two forces is 40°. Then, to find the resultant by means of the Parallelogram of Forces, we must draw two lines *PQ* and *PS* (Fig. 6) at an angle of 40° to each other, whose lengths, to a convenient scale, represent the respective magnitudes—25 lb wt and 13 lb wt—of the two forces. The parallelogram *PQRS* is completed, and the diagonal *PR* drawn. Then the direction of *PR* represents the *direction* of the resultant force on the trolley, and the length of *PR* its *magnitude*. From Fig. 6 the resultant is a force of approx. 36 lb wt at an angle of $13\frac{1}{2}°$ to the 25 lb force.

The Parallelogram of Forces can obviously be used 'in reverse' to find one of the two component forces (considered to be unknown), given the resultant force and the other component. Thus, in the case of the trolley, we might have been told that a force of 36 lb wt was required to act along the direction of movement of the trolley, and that one

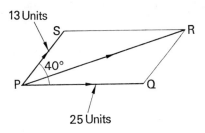

13 Units

25 Units

Fig. 6. The Parallelogram of Forces: the diagonal *PR* represents in direction and magnitude the resultant of the two forces *PS* and *PQ*.

helper was providing a pull of 25 lb wt at an angle of $13\frac{1}{2}°$ to this direction. To obtain the magnitude and direction of the second force we can draw to scale the force *PQ* and the required resultant *PR* (Fig. 6). Joining *QR* and completing the parallelogram *PQRS* then gives *PS*, which represents the required second force in both magnitude and direction.

EXERCISES

1. Explain briefly how the resultant of two forces acting at a point can be found.
2. A body is acted on by two forces, one of 5 gm wt and the other of 3 gm wt, the angle between the two forces being 120°. Find the magnitude of the resultant force (to the nearest 0·1 gm) and the angle which its direction makes (to the nearest degree) with the force of 5 gm wt.
3. Two radiographers pull along a mobile X-ray machine. They each hold the same handle, their arms being horizontal with an angle between them of 30°. If they each exert a force of 20 lb wt on the machine, what is the resultant force on the latter (answer to the nearest lb wt), and what is the direction of the resultant relative to the two applied forces?

Splitting a Given Force into Components—Rectangular Components

We have seen that two forces acting simultaneously on a body can be replaced by a single 'resultant' force, equivalent in every way to the two given forces acting together. It follows that the reverse must be possible: i.e. a single given force can be replaced by *two* separate forces which, acting simultaneously, are equivalent in every respect to the single given force. This process is known as *resolving* the given force into *components*. Consider the force represented by the line *AB* in Fig. 7. It follows from the Parallelogram of Forces that if *any* parallelogram such as *APBQ* is drawn, having *AB* as diagonal, then the lines *AP* and *AQ* represent a pair of forces which, acting simultaneously, are equivalent to the given force *AB*, i.e. they represent *components* of *AB*. Now *any number* of parallelograms can be drawn having *AB* as a diagonal: the dotted lines in Fig. 7 show a second one *AYBX*. It

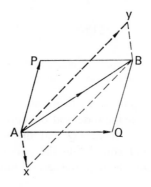

Fig. 7. *AP* and *AQ* represent *components* of the force represented by *AB*; so also do *AY* and *AX*.

follows that there are *any number* of pairs of components equivalent to a single given force. (This is in contrast to the combination of two given forces into a single resultant—which can be done in one way only, i.e. two given forces acting at a point have only a single resultant.)

Thus, when replacing a given force by two components equivalent to it, it seems that we are faced with an unlimited choice. In a practical problem, however, there are usually conditions which have to be fulfilled which determine the pair of components actually chosen. By far the commonest case is the replacement of the given force by two components which are required to be at right angles to each other, one of them making a stated angle with the given force. In this case the parallelogram to be drawn, in order to find the components, is the special case of a *rectangle*, and for this reason such components are called *rectangular* components.

Consider our mobile X-ray machine again, and imagine that this time one person only is pulling it along by a handle low enough to result in the force being applied at an angle of 30° to the horizontal. Then this force may be resolved into (or replaced by) a pair of components at right angles to each other, one horizontal, and the other vertical. To find these components, let us suppose that the applied force is one of 50 lb wt. Then, to a convenient scale, draw *AB* (Fig. 8) to represent

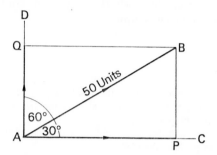

Fig. 8. *AQ* and *AP* represent two components at right angles into which the force represented by *AB* can be resolved.

the applied force in both magnitude and direction. The lines *AC* and *AD* are drawn at right angles to each other, making angles of 30° and 60° respectively with *AB*. Perpendiculars *BP*, *BQ* are drawn from *B* on to *AC* and *AD* respectively. Then *AB* is a diagonal of the rectangle *APBQ*, and *AP* and *AQ* therefore represent the required components. *AP* is found to be 43·3 lb wt and *AQ* 25 lb wt.* Thus a force of 50 lb wt applied to the machine in the described manner results in a force of 43·3 lb wt which pulls the machine along, and a force of 25 lb wt tending to *lift* the machine. By constructing a number of different rectangles it is easily seen that as the direction of *AB* approaches the horizontal the component *AP* approaches more and more closely the value of *AB* itself, whilst the component *AQ* steadily diminishes. *Thus it pays to apply the given force in such a manner that its direction approximates as closely as possible to that in which the machine is to move.*

* Students familiar with elementary trigonometry (see 'Mathematics for Radiographers', Ch. 7) will realize that, since
$$AP = AB \cos 30°,$$
and
$$AQ = AB \cos 60°,$$
the two rectangular components can easily be calculated with the aid of trigonometric tables and without the necessity of a scale drawing.

N.B. When a given force is split into two rectangular components, each of these components is often referred to as the *resolved part* of the given force in that particular direction, because each rectangular component represents the *whole effect* of the given force *in that direction*. This is perhaps more obvious when it is realized that neither component can contribute towards movement in the direction of the other when the components are at right angles to each other. For example, in the case discussed above, the vertical component contributes nothing towards moving the machine along.

EXERCISES

1. A trolley is *pushed* along by a force of 30 lb wt inclined *downwards* at an angle of 20° to the horizontal. What is the resolved part of the force in (a) the horizontal direction, and (b) the vertical direction (to nearest lb wt)? What functions do these components perform?
2. Repeat Ex. 1 for the same force but applied at an angle of 40°.Which represents the better way of pushing the trolley?

PIVOTED OBJECTS—THE MOMENT OF A FORCE

So far, we have been discussing the action of forces on objects free to move bodily from one place to another. There are many examples of bodies which are not free to move in this way, but which, being *pivoted*, are capable of *rotary* movement. In this case it is convenient to give special consideration to the *turning effect* which a force applied to such a body may have.

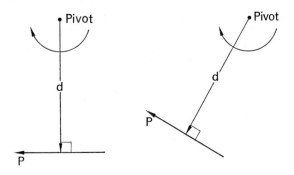

Fig. 9. The turning *moment* of the force *P* about the pivot is given by the product *d.P.*

Many rotary mechanisms are operated manually by means of a handle at the end of a crank (or attached near the edge of a wheel), the handle being pushed round by a force whose direction is being changed continuously so as to maintain it at right angles to the arm of the crank (Fig. 9). Common examples are the handle of a winch and the starting handles of cars. Some students may also have used X-ray machines in which the tube is raised and lowered by a handle rotated in the manner described. Consider a force P applied in this way to a crank handle, the length of whose arm is d ft (Fig. 9). It is well known that the turning effect of the force will depend partly on the length of the arm of the crank, as well as on the magnitude of the force: the *longer* the arm, the *greater* the turning effect of the force. (For this reason the starting handle of a large lorry has to have a much longer arm than the starting handle of a small car.) Combining the effects of both the arm length and the magnitude of the force, the turning effect (known as the *moment* of the force about the given axis of rotation) can be represented by the *product* $d.P$ (Fig. 9). Note again that the force is applied in such a way that its direction is always at right angles to the arm.

The Principle of Moments

Consider a plank pivoted at its midpoint so as to serve as a see-saw (Fig. 10). Suppose an adult of weight 150 lb sits on one side and a child of weight 50 lb on the other side. Then, unless some careful

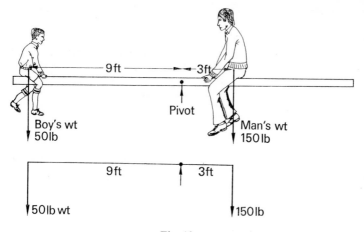

Fig. 10.

adjustment of position is made, the adult's greater weight will cause the see-saw to tilt. It is common knowledge that the balance can be restored if the adult moves *nearer the pivot*. In the particular case considered, in which the adult is 3 times heavier than the child, the weights are found to balance each other when the distance of the child from the pivot is 3 times that of the adult. Suppose the two distances are 9 ft and 3 ft respectively. Then the force represented by the child's weight has a *moment* of (50 × 9) units about the pivot, and is tending to turn the see-saw *anti*-clockwise, whilst the force represented by the adult's weight has a moment of (150 × 3) units about the pivot, and is tending to turn the see-saw *clockwise*.

Now (50 × 9) is equal to (150 × 3), and, generalizing, we may draw the following conclusion: *when a pivoted body is acted on by two forces, one of which is tending to turn it clockwise and the other to turn it anti-clockwise, and the body is balanced, then the clockwise moment is equal to the anti-clockwise moment.*

This result can easily be extended to cover the case of two children on the same side but at different distances from the pivot, balanced by one adult on the other side. In these circumstances, the sum of the moments of the weights of the two children must be equal to the moment of the adult's weight.

This principle may be stated as follows: *when a pivoted body acted on by a number of forces (some of which are tending to turn it clockwise, and some anti-clockwise) is balanced, then the sum of the moments of the forces tending to turn the body clockwise is equal to the sum of the moments of the forces tending to turn the body anti-clockwise.*

EXAMPLE

A metre rule is pivoted at its mid-point, and weights of 60 gm and 50 gm are suspended on one side of the pivot at distances of 40 cm and 20 cm respectively.

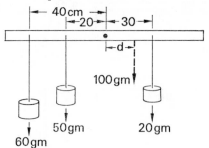

Fig. 11

On the other side a 20 gm weight is suspended at 30 cm from the pivot (Fig. 11). Where must another weight of 100 gm be placed on this side in order to balance the metre rule?

Let the distance (from the pivot) at which the 100 gm weight must be placed be d cm.

Clockwise

    (a) moment of 20 gm weight $= (\ 20 \times 30)$ units,

    (b) moment of 100 gm weight $= (100 \times \ d\ )$ units.

Anti-clockwise

    (a) moment of 60 gm weight $= (60 \times 40)$ units,

    (b) moment of 50 gm weight $= (50 \times 20)$ units.

For balance:

sum of clockwise moments = sum of anti-clockwise moments, i.e.

$$(20 \times 30) + (100 \times d) = (60 \times 40) + (50 \times 20),$$
$$\text{or } 100 \ . \ d = 2400 + 1000 - 600,$$
$$\text{whence } d = 28 \text{ cm.}$$

EXERCISES

1. A pivoted body is acted on by a force of 50 lb wt whose distance from the pivot is 3 ft. At what distance from the pivot must a force of 30 lb wt act in order to balance the turning effect of the first force?

2. A wooden rule is pivoted at its mid-point. Two weights, one of 2 lb and the other of 3 lb, are suspended on one side of the pivot at distances from it of 2 ft and 1 ft respectively. What is the magnitude of the weight which, acting 1 ft from the pivot on the other side, will balance the rule?

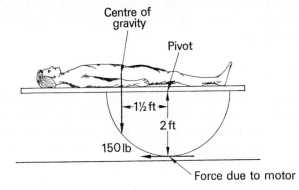

Fig. 12.

3. The weight of a patient (150 lb) lying on an X-ray couch, can be considered to act at a distance of $1\frac{1}{2}$ ft from the pivot (Fig. 12). What force (additional to that required to tilt the couch itself) must an electric motor exert at a distance of 2 ft from the pivot in order to begin tilting the patient towards the vertical?

CHAPTER 3

Dynamics—The Study of Motion

SPEED AND VELOCITY

In everyday life the words *speed* and *velocity* are employed synony-
mously to denote the rate at which a body is travelling, i.e. the distance
it travels in unit time. Thus we may refer to the speed of a train as
60 miles per hour or the speed of a man walking as 4 miles per hour,
and nothing is said about the *direction* in which the train or the man is
travelling. In fact we do not feel it necessary to make any statement
about direction when referring to the speed of anything.

On the other hand, we have already made it clear that we shall
regard *velocity* as a *vector*; that is to say, as having direction as well as
magnitude associated with it. We shall therefore make this distinction
between the two words, a distinction which is not made in everyday
language: that *speed* denotes merely the rate at which a body is travelling and has nothing to say about the direction (i.e. it is a *scalar* having
magnitude only), whereas velocity has in addition the idea of direction
associated with it.

Average Speed

A train may perform a certain journey, of, say, 200 miles in 4 hours,
and there may be many changes of speed and a number of stops
during the journey. The *average* speed is the steady or constant speed
at which the train would have to travel in order to cover the same
journey in the same time. Clearly,

$$\text{average speed} = \frac{\text{total distance}}{\text{total time taken}}.$$

∴ in above example, average speed $= \dfrac{200}{4} = 50$ mph.

Conversely, if we are told that a man maintains an average speed of

3 mph when walking, we can find how far he goes in a given time by multiplying the average speed by the time, i.e.

distance = average speed × time.

Thus in 5 hours a man walking at an average speed of 3 mph covers a distance of 15 miles.

EXERCISES

1. Distinguish between speed and velocity.
2. Define average speed.
   The average speed of a train is 45 mph. How long will it take to do a journey of 157½ miles?
3. On a journey a man walks 5 miles along a flat road in 1½ hr and 1 mile uphill in ½ hr. What is his average speed?

Graph of Distance against Time for a Body Travelling at Constant Speed

If a body is travelling at constant speed, then, for equal amounts added to the time of travel, equal amounts will be added to the distance it has travelled. This means that the graph of distance against time will be a *straight line*. Further, since at zero time the distance travelled will also be zero, the line will pass through the origin.

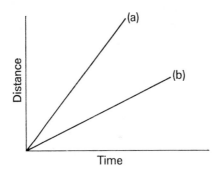

Fig. 13. Graphs of distance against time for two bodies travelling at different constant speeds.

If one body is travelling at a greater speed than another, the graph of distance against time for the faster body will be *steeper* than the corresponding graph for the slower one. Thus in Fig. 13 the graph (a) corresponds to a body moving at a greater speed than the body to which graph (b) relates.

Graph of Speed against Time for a Body Travelling at Constant Speed

If the speed of a body is constant, then its value at any particular moment will be the same as at any other moment, and the graph of speed (Fig. 14) against time will be a *straight line*, parallel to the time axis.

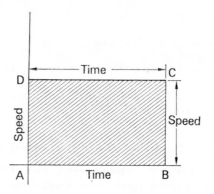

Fig. 14. Graph of speed against time for a body travelling at constant speed.

To obtain the distance travelled in a given time by a body moving at constant speed, we multiply the speed by the time. In Fig. 14, let *AB* represent the given time. If, then, the rectangle *ABCD* be drawn, *BC* can be taken to represent the speed, and we have

$$
\begin{aligned}
\text{distance} &= \text{speed} \times \text{time} \\
&= AB \times BC \\
&= \text{area of rectangle } ABCD.
\end{aligned}
$$

Putting it into words, we may say that the distance travelled by the body in a given time is represented by the *area* of the rectangle *ABCD* under the speed-time graph, in which *AB* (or *DC*) represents the given time, and *BC* (or *AD*) the speed at which the body is travelling.*

ACCELERATION

When the throttle of a car is opened, the car gathers speed: it is said to *accelerate*. If the speedometer of the car is read at the end of each

---

* There will be other occasions where we shall find that a consideration of the area under a graph yields interesting information.

second from the start, the readings might be 2 mph, 4 mph, 6 mph, 8 mph, 10 mph, and so on; that is, in every second, the speed of the car increases by 2 mph. In fact, we say that the acceleration of the car is 2 mph *every second*, or simply 2 mph *per sec*. Acceleration therefore measures the *rate of change of speed*. We might tabulate the data as follows:

Time	0	1	2	3	4	5	6	. . . etc., sec
Speed	0	2	4	6	8	10	12	. . . etc., mph

Acceleration (rate of change of speed) = 2 mph every sec.
$$= 2 \text{ mph } per\ sec.$$
Or (since 2 mph = 2·9 ft per sec) we may write,
$$\text{acceleration} = 2\cdot9 \text{ ft per sec. per sec.}$$
Thus the rather clumsy phrase 'ft per sec per sec' need not cause undue concern. It means simply that in every second the speed of the car increases by 2·9 ft per sec, i.e. after one sec its speed is 2·9 ft per sec, after 2 sec its speed is 5·8 ft per sec, after 3 sec it is 8·7 ft per sec and so on. What might be termed a mathematical shorthand device is often used to avoid the clumsiness of the phrase: the fact that 'per sec' occurs twice in succession is indicated by writing simply 'per sec²'. Thus an acceleration of so many ft per sec per sec is written simply as so many ft per $\sec^2$. It must be remembered, however, that this shorthand trick has nothing to do with multiplying anything by itself!

In a similar manner, in the Metric system of units, we have accelerations expressed as so many cm per sec per sec, or simply cm per $\sec^2$.

In all that we have said so far we have assumed the change of speed to be the same in each second. In fact we have assumed the *acceleration* to be *constant* or *uniform*, and we shall confine our attention to accelerations of this type; that is to say, we shall *not* consider motion where the acceleration itself is subject to changes.

Deceleration or Retardation

Suppose the engine of a car running at 30 mph is switched off, and the brakes are applied. The speedometer readings taken every second from the moment the engine was switched off might now be as follows:

Time	0	1	2	3	4	5	6	sec
Speed	30	25	20	15	10	5	0	mph

In this case the car is slowing down: it is being *retarded* at a constant rate of 5 mph every second. It is said to have a *deceleration* or *retardation* of 5 mph per sec or 7·3 ft per sec per sec. Since deceleration or retardation is the opposite of acceleration, it is often called a *negative acceleration*. In fact, problems involving deceleration can be worked out in exactly the same way as problems on acceleration, if a negative sign is given to the value of the deceleration.

EXAMPLES

1. A car possessing a uniform acceleration attains a speed from rest of 60 mph in 22 sec. Express its acceleration in ft per sec².

$$60 \text{ mph} = 60 \times 5280 \text{ ft } per\ hr$$
$$= \frac{60 \times 5280}{60 \times 60} \text{ ft } per\ sec.$$
$$\therefore \text{ Speed change} = \frac{60 \times 5280}{60 \times 60} \text{ ft per sec in 22 sec}$$
$$\therefore \text{ in 1 sec speed change} = \frac{60 \times 5280}{60 \times 60} \times \frac{1}{22}$$
$$= \frac{88}{22} \text{ ft per sec}$$

i.e. acceleration = 4 ft per sec per sec (4 ft per sec²).

2. An object moving at 60 metres per sec is retarded uniformly for 20 sec, at the end of which interval its speed has fallen to 40 metres per sec. What is its retardation in cm per sec²?

$$60 \text{ metres per sec} = 6000 \text{ cm per sec}$$
$$\text{and } 40 \text{ metres per sec} = 4000 \text{ cm per sec}$$
$$\therefore \text{ change of speed in 20 sec} = 2000 \text{ cm per sec}$$
$$\text{i.e. change of speed in 1 sec} = \frac{2000}{20} \text{ cm per sec}$$
$$= 100 \text{ cm per sec}$$

Hence, retardation = 100 cm per sec per sec (100 cm per sec²).

EXERCISES

1. Define acceleration and retardation. In what units are they commonly measured?
2. What is. meant by *uniform* acceleration? The speedometer of a car is read at 1 sec intervals. The readings are as follows:

Time	0	1	2	3	4	5	6	sec
Speed	0	1·5	3·0	4·5	5·5	6·0	6·0	mph

Over what interval might it be stated that the car had uniform acceleration? Work out this acceleration in ft per sec².

3. An object moving at 40 cm per sec is uniformly retarded for 12 sec. If the retardation has a value of 2·5 cm per sec per sec, what is the speed of the object at the end of the interval?

Graph of Distance against Time for a Body Travelling with Uniform Acceleration

Where there is acceleration the speed will steadily increase from zero, and consequently, in successive equal intervals of time the body will travel increasing distances. The graph of distance against time thus gets steeper with increasing time, as indicated in Fig. 15. The graphs

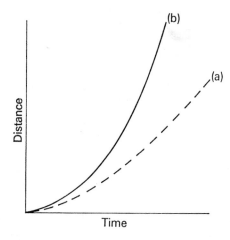

Fig. 15. Graphs of distance against time for two bodies travelling with different uniform accelerations.

corresponding to two bodies having different (uniform) accelerations will be of the same general shape (in fact parabolic), but that belonging to the body having the smaller acceleration (*a*) will lie *under* the one belonging to that with the greater acceleration (*b*).

Graph of Speed against Time for a Body Travelling with Uniform Acceleration

When a body has a uniform acceleration then, in successive equal intervals of time, equal amounts are added to its speed. It follows that the speed-time graph will in this case be a straight line (Fig. 16), and if, in addition, at zero time the speed is also zero, this straight line will pass through the origin. Where the acceleration of one body is greater than that of another, the speed-time graph (*a*) associated with it will have a steeper slope than the corresponding graph (*b*) associated with the more slowly accelerating body.

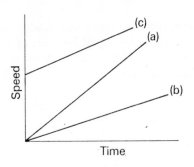

Fig. 16. Graphs of speed against time for bodies travelling with different uniform accelerations.

In the case where a body possessing uniform acceleration has an *initial* speed at the beginning of the interval of time considered, the speed-time graph will not pass through the origin, but instead will pass through a point on the speed axis representing this initial speed (*c*).

For a body moving with uniform acceleration it can easily be shown as follows that (as in the case of a body moving at constant speed, p. 20) the *area* under the speed-time graph represents the *distance* travelled.

Consider first a body starting from rest, i.e. having *zero* initial speed. Suppose that *OB* (Fig. 17) represents its speed-time graph. Then, in the time interval represented by *OA*, the average speed—which in this case is given by ½ (speed at beginning of interval + speed at end of interval)—is simply equal to half the speed at the end of the interval, since the initial speed is zero.

But *AB* represents the speed at the end of the interval, and so ½ *AB* represents the average speed.

Now,   distance = average speed × time
            = (½ *AB*) × *OA*
            = area of triangle *OAB*.

Next consider a body which has an initial speed at the beginning of the time interval considered. Suppose that CB (Fig. 17) represents its speed-time graph. Then we have,

average speed during interval $= \frac{1}{2}$ (speed at beginning of interval + speed at end of interval)
$$= \tfrac{1}{2}(OC + AB).$$
$\therefore$ distance travelled $=$ (average speed $\times$ time)
$$= \tfrac{1}{2}(OC + AB) \times OA$$
$$= \text{area of } OABC.$$

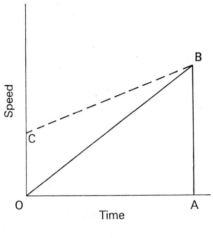

Fig. 17

Thus, in either case, we may say in words that, even when a body possesses acceleration, the area under the speed-time graph corresponding to a given time interval represents the distance travelled by the body during that time.

EQUATIONS OF UNIFORMLY ACCELERATED MOTION

It is often possible to group problems in such a way that those belonging to the same group may be worked out by applying the same general method. Thus, in problems on accelerated motion letters may be used to denote the initial speed, acceleration, distance, etc., and formulae then derived showing how, for example, the final speed may be worked

3

out if the initial speed, acceleration, and time are given. The symbols usually employed are as follows:

u, denoting initial speed,
v, ,,   final speed,
a, ,,   acceleration,
t, ,,   time,
s, ,,   distance travelled.

Equation 1

If a body has an initial speed of 10 ft per sec and an acceleration of 3 ft per sec², then after 5 sec its speed will have been increased by (3 × 5) ft per sec, and its final speed will therefore be 10 + (3 × 5) ft per sec. Similarly, if a body has an initial speed of u, and an aceleration a, then in time t its speed will have been increased by (a × t) and the final speed will be ($u + at$).

$$\text{i.e.} \qquad v = u + at. \qquad (1)$$

Note that if the body starts from rest, $u = 0$,

$$\text{and} \qquad v = at. \qquad (1a)$$

It is important to realize that when substituting the values of the letters in such formulae, care must be taken to use consistent units. Thus, in the case of the above formulae, if the final speed is in ft per sec and the time in sec, it would be quite wrong, for instance, to put the initial speed in mph, the acceleration in ft per sec² and the time in minutes!

EXERCISES

1. A car travelling at 10 mph is accelerated for 7 sec at the rate of $1\frac{1}{2}$ mph per sec. What is its new speed?
2. The brakes of a vehicle standing on a hill are released, and the vehicle runs down, accelerating uniformly for 24 sec. Its speed is then found to be 18 mph. What was the acceleration to which it was subject?
3. A moving vehicle is accelerated uniformly at a rate of 2 mph per sec for 9 sec. Its speed is then 23 mph. What was its speed prior to the period of acceleration?

Equation 2

This may be derived simply by expressing in symbols the fact that

$$\text{distance} = \text{average speed} \times \text{time}.$$

As we have already noted (p. 24), when the acceleration is constant, the average speed is equal to

$\frac{1}{2}$ (initial speed + final speed) $= \dfrac{u + v}{2}$.

Thus, distance $s = \left(\dfrac{u + v}{2}\right) t.$ (2)

If the body starts from rest, $u = 0$, and in this case

$$s = \frac{vt}{2}.$$ (2a)

EXERCISES

1. A lift starts from rest and accelerates uniformly for 3 sec, when its speed becomes constant at 6 ft per sec. How far has it travelled in this time?
2. A car travelling at 30 ft per sec changes its speed at a uniform rate to 20 ft per sec in 3 sec. How far does it travel in this time?
3. A train starts from rest and with uniform acceleration reaches a speed of 50 ft per sec in 20 sec. It then runs at constant speed for 5 min, after which it *de*celerates uniformly, to come to rest in 10 sec. What is the length of its journey (in feet)?

Equation 3

This is obtained by combining equations (1) and (2) in such a way that we obtain a formula enabling us to calculate the *distance*, when we are given the initial velocity, the acceleration and the time.

Thus, $s = \left(\dfrac{u + v}{2}\right) t.$ (Eq. 2)

But from, Eq. (1), $v = (u + at)$,
and we may therefore substitute $(u + at)$ for v in Eq. (2).

Hence, $s = \dfrac{u + (u + at)}{2} \cdot t$

$= \dfrac{2u + at}{2} \cdot t,$

i.e. $s = ut + \frac{1}{2}at^2.$ (3)

If the initial velocity is zero, then $s = \frac{1}{2}at^2.$ (3a)

EXAMPLES

1. How far will a vehicle travel in 10 sec if its initial velocity is 5 ft per sec, and it has a uniform acceleration of 4 ft per sec^2?

$$u = 5 \text{ ft per sec}$$
$$a = 4 \text{ ft per sec}^2$$
$$t = 10 \text{ sec}$$
$$\therefore \text{ distance } s = ut + \tfrac{1}{2}at^2$$
$$= (5 \times 10) + (\tfrac{1}{2} \times 4 \times 10^2)$$
$$= 250 \text{ ft.}$$

2. An object has an initial speed of 150 cm per sec, and slows up for 6 sec as the result of a uniform deceleration. The distance travelled during this time is 540 cm. What is the deceleration in cm per sec^2?

$$u = 150 \text{ cm per sec}$$
$$t = 6 \text{ sec}$$
$$s = 540 \text{ cm}$$

$\therefore$ since $\qquad s = ut + \tfrac{1}{2}at^2,$

we have $\qquad 540 = (150 \times 6) + (\tfrac{1}{2} \times 6^2 \times a).$

i.e. $\qquad 540 - 900 = 18a,$

or $\qquad a = -20 \text{ cm per sec}^2.$

EXERCISES

1. A car starts from rest with uniform acceleration, and travels a distance of 400 ft in 20 sec. What is its acceleration?
2. A train takes 15 sec to come to rest. How far will it travel in this time if it has a deceleration of 4 ft per sec^2 and at the moment of applying the brakes its speed is 60 ft per sec?
3. What time will an object take to travel 22 cm if its initial speed is 7 cm per sec, and it is subject to an acceleration of 4 cm per sec^2?

Equation 4

Since $\qquad v = u + at$ $\hfill$ (Eq. 1)

$$v^2 = (u + at)^2$$
$$= u^2 + 2uat + a^2t^2.$$

This may be written as follows:

$$v^2 = u^2 + 2a(ut + \tfrac{1}{2}at^2),$$

(easily verified by removing the brackets).

Now the quantity inside the bracket in the last equation is equal to s (see Eq. 3), and hence,

$$v^2 = u^2 + 2as. \hfill (4)$$

If the initial velocity is zero,

$$v^2 = 2as. \hfill (4a)$$

These equations indicate how we may work out the final velocity if we are given the initial velocity, the acceleration, and the distance.

EXERCISES

1. An object with an acceleration of 10 cm per sec² travels a distance of 500 cm. What is its velocity at the end of this interval if it started from rest?
2. What distance will be required for a car to accelerate from 15 ft per sec to 25 ft per sec if its acceleration is 2 ft per sec²?
3. What is the deceleration of a train which comes to rest in 1200 ft, its speed when the brakes were applied being 60 ft per sec.?

Summary of the Equations of Uniformly Accelerated Motion

1.
$$v = u + at.$$

2.
$$s = \left(\frac{u + v}{2} \right) t.$$

3.
$$s = ut + \tfrac{1}{2}at^2.$$

4.
$$v^2 = u^2 + 2as.$$

N.B. As already noted, for *retardations* a *minus* sign must be given to the value of a in these equations.

MOTION UNDER GRAVITY

The early Greek philosophers were much more ready to form *opinions* about scientific matters than they were to put them to the test, and so great was their reputation as philosophers that many of these opinions remained unchallenged by experiment for hundreds of years. Thus Aristotle maintained that a large weight fell through a given distance more quickly than a small weight, and this was accepted as being the case until Galileo, imbued with the true scientific spirit, decided to put Aristotle's opinion to the test by dropping a large and a small weight simultaneously from the top of the Leaning Tower of Pisa. He had called an assembly of scholars together to witness the experiment, and although the two weights reached the ground together, thus proving Aristotle to be wrong, so great was the prejudice that the assembly ignored the results of the experiment and persecuted Galileo for his views.

Since Galileo's time it has become a well-established fact that the rate at which a body falls is independent of its weight, provided that the various forms of friction do not interfere. Thus a sheet of paper will not fall as quickly as a lump of metal because of the greater effect of air friction on the paper's motion. If, however, a piece of paper and a lump of metal are allowed to fall down a glass tube from which the air has been evacuated, the two are seen to fall together.

Now it can be shown by a variety of experiments that any body falling freely under the action of gravity possesses a *constant acceleration* the value of which in British units is approximately 32 ft per sec², or 9·81 m per sec² in the Metric system. This is termed the *acceleration due to gravity*, and, since motion under gravity is one of constant acceleration, problems concerning such motion may be solved by applying the formulae derived above. In such cases it is usual to write *g* in place of *a* in the formulae, to denote the special value which the acceleration has where free fall under gravity is concerned. Note that bodies projected vertically *upwards* have a *retardation* of 32 ft per sec² or 9·81 m per sec², and in such cases *g* must be given a *minus* sign in the formulae.

EXAMPLES

1. How fast (in m per sec) will an object be travelling after falling freely from rest for 5 sec?
   The formula we require is $v = gt$
   $$\text{where} \quad g = 9\cdot81 \text{ m per sec}^2$$
   ∴ final velocity $\quad v = 9\cdot81 \times 5$
   $$= 49\cdot05 \text{ m per sec.}$$

2. A stone is dropped into a well and hits the water after 3 sec. How deep is the well?
   The implication of the statement that the stone is *dropped* is that $u = 0$. The required equation is therefore
   $$s = \tfrac{1}{2} gt^2$$
   $$\text{where } g = 9\cdot81 \text{ m per sec}^2$$
   $$\text{and } t = 3 \text{ sec.}$$
   $$\therefore \quad s = \tfrac{1}{2} \times 9\cdot81 \times 3^2$$
   $$= 44\cdot15 \text{ m}$$

EXERCISES

1. How long will a stone take to reach the sea, if it is dropped over a 100 m cliff?
2. At what speed will this stone strike the water?
3. An object is thrown vertically upwards with an initial velocity of 24·5 m per sec.

How high does it go? What is its velocity when it has fallen back to the thrower? (There is a *de*celeration, i.e. $-g$. Note also that at the highest point the velocity is momentarily zero.)

NEWTON'S LAWS OF MOTION

These laws—three in number—are among the most important of all those formulated to describe the behaviour of matter, and were put forward by the famous English scientist Isaac Newton.

Newton's First Law of Motion

Reference has already been made to the fact that inanimate matter does not move, or change its direction or speed if already moving, *of its own accord*. This is often called the principle of the Inertia of Matter, and is one way of stating Newton's First Law of Motion. Put formally, the latter states that a body continues in its state of rest or uniform motion in a straight line, except in so far as it is compelled to change that state by the application of an external force. There are many examples of this principle which are a matter of common experience. If one alights from a fast-moving vehicle one is in danger of falling over. This is because one's feet are brought rapidly to a standstill by contact with the ground, whilst the upper part of one's body tends to continue moving. The remedy is not to alight until the speed of the vehicle has dropped to such an extent that one is able to keep pace with it after alighting. One is then able gradually to reduce the speed of the body as a whole to zero. The fact that a horseman is likely to be 'thrown' over the horse's head if the horse stops suddenly is another example of the 'inertia' of matter.

Newton's Second Law of Motion

We have seen in both this chapter and the previous one that a 'force' is the means by which the inertia of matter can be overcome. Thus a stationary body may be set in motion if a *force* is applied to it; and the speed of a body already moving may be altered in a similar way. In both cases acceleration is present. This is obviously so in the latter case, for change of speed *constitutes* acceleration. In the former case, also, the force imparts an acceleration, for a body at rest must be subject to an acceleration if it is to be set in motion. Thus an alternative definition of what is meant by a force might be, that it is the agent by which *acceleration* is produced.

Newton's Second Law of Motion is concerned with the relation between a force and the acceleration produced by it. We shall not attempt to consider the law in the form in which it was put forward by Newton. Instead, we shall discuss a simple and extremely important relationship to which it leads.

Now, it is a matter of common experience that a *massive* body is more difficult to set in motion than a light one; and that to impart the same speed to it in a given time requires the application of a bigger force. This is only another way of saying that the acceleration produced by a force depends on the *mass* of the body on which it acts (i.e. the amount of *matter* in it).

If we talk about retardations instead of accelerations, the truth of this is perhaps even more easily recognized, for clearly a massive body is much more difficult to stop in a given time (i.e. it requires a much larger force) than a light one initially moving at the same speed. In short, the force acting, the mass of the body on which it acts, and the acceleration produced, are inter-related. The relationship between these three quantities may be deduced from Newton's Second Law of Motion, and provided that special units are used in which to denote the magnitude of the force, then the relationship may be stated very simply as follows:

$$force = mass \times acceleration.$$

The general truth of this equation is easily seen from the above discussion.

The unit of force which must be employed in this equation is clearly that which, acting on unit mass, produces unit acceleration; for, then, on substitution, we have

1 (unit of force) = 1 (unit of mass) $\times$ 1 (unit of acceleration).

In the Metric system the new absolute unit of force is that which produces an acceleration of 1 m per sec^2 when it acts on a mass of 1 kgm. This is called the newton (N). The older Metric unit, to which reference will still often be found, is the *dyne*, corresponding to the force which, acting on a mass of 1 gm, produces an acceleration of 1 cm per sec^2. It is clear, therefore, that *one newton* is equal to 10^5 dynes.

In Chapter II, the gravitational unit of force, the *gramme-weight*, was used, representing the force due to gravity on a mass of one gramme. From the equation:

$$\text{force} = \text{mass} \times \text{acceleration},$$
$$1 \text{ gm wt} = 10^{-3} \text{ kgm} \times 9\cdot81 \text{ m per sec}^2,$$
$$= 9\cdot81 \times 10^{-3} \text{ newtons},$$
$$= 981 \text{ dynes.*}$$

It is important that in applying this equation a consistent set of units is used:

	New system	Old system
Force	newtons	dynes
Mass	kilogrammes	grammes
Acceleration	metres per sec²	cm per sec²

EXAMPLES

1. A mass of $1\frac{1}{2}$ kgm, travelling at 1 m per sec, is brought to rest in 5 sec by a certain force. What is the value of the latter (in newtons)?
The acceleration must first be found.

We have $\quad v = u + at,$
where $\quad v = 0$
$\quad u = 1 \text{ (m per sec)}$
and $\quad t = 5 \text{ (sec)}.$

Hence, by substitution,
$$a = -0\cdot2 \text{ m per sec}^2.$$

Then, force (in newtons) $= \text{mass (in kgm)} \times \text{acceleration (in m per sec}^2)$
$$= 1\cdot5 \times (-0\cdot2)$$
$$= -0\cdot3$$

that is, a retarding force of 0·3 newton.

2. A portion (the nucleus of a hydrogen atom, see p. 91) of mass $\frac{5}{3} \times 10^{-24}$ gm is acted on by an electric field which produces on it a force of 5×10^{-12} dynes. What acceleration is produced, and what would be the proton's speed in 1/10,000 sec. if it started from rest?†

---

* In the British system of units, the unit of force is the *poundal*, the force which produces an acceleration of 1 ft per sec² when acting on a mass of one pound. The gravitational unit, the pound weight (p. 7), is then equal to 32 poundals as the acceleration due to gravity is 32 ft per sec² (p. 30).

† When particles travel at speeds approaching that of light, the theory of *Relativity* shows that Newton's Laws must be modified. All the examples in this book have been selected to avoid this complication.

Force (in dynes) = mass (in gm) × acceleration (in cm per sec^2),

or $5 \times 10^{-12} = \dfrac{5}{3} \times 10^{-24} \times a$.

$$\therefore a = \dfrac{5 \times 10^{-12}}{\frac{5}{3} \times 10^{-24}}$$

$$= 3 \times 10^{12} \text{ cm per sec}^2.$$

Thus in 1/10,000 sec (after starting from rest) the velocity v is given by:

$$v = at,$$

$$= 3 \times 10^{12} \times \dfrac{1}{10,000}$$

$$= 3 \times 10^9 \text{ cm per sec}$$

(i.e. approximately 2000 miles per sec).

EXERCISES

1. A force of 5 newtons acts on a mass of 10 kgm. What acceleration results?
2. An object of 3·5 kgm is acted on by a certain force, which, after the object has travelled 5 cm from rest, has generated a velocity of 10 cm per sec. What is the value of the force (in newtons)? (N.B. First use $v^2 = 2as$ to find a).
3. A deuteron (a 'heavy' hydrogen nucleus) has a mass of approximately $3\frac{1}{3} \times 10^{-24}$ gm. Under the accelerating force due to a certain electric field, it takes 1/500 sec to travel 10 cm starting from rest. What is the force acting on it (in dynes), and what is the final velocity?

Newton's Third Law of Motion

This law is concerned with the fact that the action of bodies on one another by means of forces is *mutual*. This means that if one body produces a certain force on another, then one may say at once that the second body is producing an equal and opposite force on the first. Newton called the first force the *action* and the force which it calls into play *reaction*, and his Third Law of Motion states that action and reaction are equal and opposite.

Some examples of this law are obvious enough and easy to understand, whilst others are a little perplexing on first acquaintance. An obvious example is that of one object supported by another on which it rests, for instance a book on a table. The book exerts a force equal to its own weight on the table, and an equal and opposite force is called into play, namely the force which is exerted on the book *by the table*, balancing the weight of the book and preventing it from falling.

Gravitational attraction between two bodies is a rather less obvious example. We are familiar with the fact that the earth exerts a force of attraction on other bodies, but we do not find it so easy to realize that the attraction is a mutual one, and that whilst it is true that the earth exerts a force of attraction on a body (which we call its weight), the body concerned exerts an equal and opposite force on the earth. The effect of this force on the earth is imperceptible in the case of terrestrial objects, on account of the enormous mass of the earth compared with that of any objects with which we deal on the earth's surface. When, however, we consider an object whose mass is of the same order as, or much greater than, that of the earth, the mutual nature of the attraction becomes evident. Thus the earth exerts a gravitational attraction on the moon, and it is this which constrains the moon to move round the earth in a closed path instead of pursuing a straight course through space in accordance with the principle of inertia. The fact that there is a reciprocal force exerted by the moon on the earth is demonstrated by the way in which the vast quantities of water constituting the seas respond to this attraction, producing the tides.

An even less obvious example is the fact that any surface (e.g. the floor) exerts a forward force on our feet as we walk, being the reaction to the backward force exerted on the surface by our feet. A moment's thought will make it obvious that this forward force must be present, and that it is this force which is responsible for our forward movement.

EXAMPLE

Give an account of the variations which occur in the reaction between the floor of a lift and the feet of a person travelling in it.

(a) Suppose the lift starts from rest on an *upward* journey. To begin with (i.e. before the lift starts) the reaction is simply equal and opposite to the person's weight. When the lift begins to move upwards there is an initial period of acceleration, after which the lift travels with uniform velocity for a certain time before being brought to rest. During the acceleration the person in the lift is subject to the same acceleration as the lift, and the reaction between the person's feet and the lift floor must *increase* by an amount equal to the force required to produce this acceleration in a mass equal to that of the person. (One is made conscious of this additional force by the tendency of one's knees to bend as the lift starts up.) When the acceleration ceases, this additional force vanishes, and during the period of uniform velocity the reaction is once again equal simply to the weight of the passenger. As the lift is brought to rest, it (and its passenger) is subject to a *de*celeration, with the result that the reaction between the passenger's feet and the lift floor *decreases* by an amount equal to the force necessary to produce this deceleration.

(b) For a downward journey, the above variations occur in the reverse order. Thus, during the initial acceleration downwards there is a decrease in the reaction, followed by a period of uniform velocity during which the reaction is equal to its stationary value, and finally a period of deceleration (opposite in direction to the one referred to under (a)) during which the reaction is increased. It is perhaps an academic point, but worth noting, that if the lift broke away and fell freely under gravity, the passenger inside would also be falling freely under gravity, and the reaction between feet and floor would vanish!

MOMENTUM

We have already noted in connection with Newton's Second Law that the ease with which an object can be brought to rest depends on its mass. It obviously depends also on the velocity with which it is moving. The product (mass × velocity) is called the *momentum* of the body.

Momentum has sometimes been described as a measure of the amount of 'motion' possessed by a moving object. Thus an object with a lot of 'motion' (momentum) is much less easily stopped than one with a small amount of 'motion'. When used in this sense, the word *motion* should not be confused with speed (or velocity): for a light object travelling fast (e.g. a paper pellet) may be much more easily stopped than a heavy object (e.g. a loaded railway goods truck) moving much more slowly. This is because momentum equals (mass × velocity), and a large mass may more than compensate for a small velocity. Thus, in collisions at sea, the damage may be very considerable (even though the speed of the ships is low) because in this case the masses involved are extremely large.

Momentum is a Vector

Momentum is the product of a scalar (mass) and a vector (velocity) and as such it has *direction* (that of the velocity) and is itself a *vector*. This is important in the discussion which follows.

Conservation of Momentum

There are many important instances of the fact that when two objects interact (e.g. collide) with one another, they are found to possess the same *total* momentum *after* interacting as they possessed *before* doing so. This is actually a consequence of Newton's Third Law of Motion.

Consider a head-on collision between a moving object and one initially stationary. These two objects might be two billiard balls, or two atomic particles, such as a fast-moving *neutron* (an atomic particle without electrical charge) which 'strikes' the stationary *nucleus* (p. 91) of an atom (excluding the cases where a *nuclear reaction* results, when, obviously, the collision can no longer be treated as a simple mechanical one).

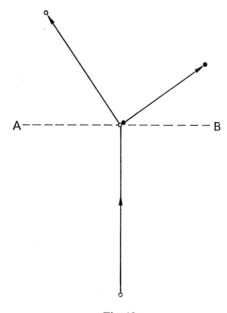

Fig. 18.

At each and every instant during the time of interaction (which may be, and often will be, very short) the object initially moving produces a force (the 'action') on the object struck, and the latter produces an equal and opposite force (the 'reaction') on the object which has collided with it. As a result of the collision, the stationary object is set in motion, and the moving object is slowed down (it may, in some circumstances, even be brought to rest), and by an application of Newton's Second Law of Motion it can easily be shown that the momentum *gained* by the struck object is equal to the momentum *lost* by the object striking it, i.e. momentum is *conserved* during the collision.

It is very important to realize that since momentum is a vector quantity, directions of motion (both before and after collision) must be given full consideration in applying the Law of Conservation of Momentum.

Head-on collision is simple: the momentum gained by the struck object has the same direction as that lost by the object which strikes it, and numerically the magnitudes of the momenta gained and lost are equal.

In oblique collision, however (Fig. 18), we must apply the Principle of the Conservation of Momentum *twice over*, in effect first stating that the *total* momentum of the two objects in the initial direction of the moving one is *unchanged* (as for head-on collision), and secondly, that the total momentum in a direction *at right angles to this is also unchanged, being zero both before and after collision.**

WORK

If resistance to motion could be eliminated altogether, then a body, once set moving, would go on for ever without needing any further application of a force to keep it in motion (Newton's First Law, p. 31). But resistance cannot be entirely eliminated. Thus, if the motion of a body is such that some component of its movement is in the upward direction, then its *own weight* (i.e. the force of gravity on it) offers a resistance to the movement. Even if the motion is horizontal (so that there is no question of overcoming gravity), there will be resistance to motion, for no surfaces can be made absolutely smooth, nor can they be perfectly lubricated. Consequently, whenever one surface slides over another, some resistance to motion is present. This is called *friction*, and mechanical effort must be expended (that is, a force must be applied) to overcome it if motion is to be maintained.

Whenever a force is applied in order to produce motion against a resistance (due to friction, gravitational attraction, the force of repulsion between electric charges or to the presence of other fields of

* This follows from the fact that no vector has any component in a direction at right angles to itself (p. 14) and thus there is no nett momentum in either direction along *AB* (Fig. 18) before the collision. After collision the two objects move off obliquely as shown, and it follows that if the total momentum in the direction *AB* is still to be zero, then, after collision, the *resolved part* of the momentum of the first object along the line of *AB* must be *equal and opposite* to the resolved part of the momentum of the second object along the same line.

force), the force (and therefore, ultimately, the agent generating it) has to do *work*. The amount of work done depends on two things: on the *magnitude* of the force which has to be exerted to maintain motion, and on the distance moved. The work done by a force of one *newton* when the point at which it is applied moves a distance of one *metre in the direction of the force*, is called one *joule*. The corresponding unit of work for a force of one *dyne* acting over a distance of one centimetre is referred to as an *erg*. A simple calculation then shows that one joule is equivalent to 10^7 ergs. It is clear, therefore, that in order to find the work done by a force when it produces a certain movement *in its own direction* we must multiply the distance by the magnitude of the force. That is:

$$work = force \times distance.$$

EXAMPLE

Calculate the work done against gravity in raising a mass of 500 gm vertically through a distance of 1·5 metres.

To *lift* an object, one must overcome the force due to gravity. This force is given by:

force (in newtons) = mass (in kgm) ×
acceleration (in m per sec²)
= 0·5 × 9·81 = 4·91.

The movement is vertical, that is in the direction of the applied force overcoming the gravitational attraction, so that:

work done = force (in newtons) × distance moved (in metres)
= 4·91 × 1·5
= 7·36 joules.

It is important to realize that a force can be applied in such a way that the motion produced is *not* in its own direction. For instance in the example on page 13, a force of 50 lb wt inclined at an angle of 30° to the horizontal is applied to an X-ray machine in order to move it along. Thus the direction of movement is at an angle of 30° to the force producing it. In such a case, the work done must be found by multiplying the distance not by the force, but by its *resolved component* in the direction of the movement.

Consider now the situation shown in Fig. 19 where a mass of 51 kgm is pushed up a plane inclined at 30° to the horizontal. It is assumed that friction is negligible, so that work is only done against gravity. For simplicity, the force is assumed to be applied in a direction parallel to the inclined plane (Fig. 19a).

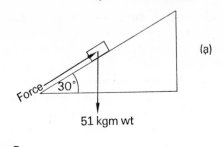

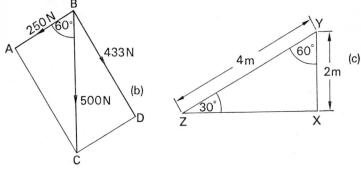

Fig. 19.

The weight of the body, that is the force due to gravity acting on this mass, is equivalent to 500 newtons (see p. 33). This force (*BC* in Fig. 19b) may be resolved into two components, *BA* acting *down* the plane and *BD* acting at right-angles into the plane. Now it is the former component force which must be overcome in order to move the body up the plane. The latter component merely serves to press the body against the plane and (in the absence of friction), being at right angles to the direction of motion does not affect it.

From the scale diagram in Fig. 19b it appears that the force acting down the plane is 250 newtons.* Thus, a force equal and opposite to this must be applied *up* the plane to produce the required movement. If the body is moved a distance of 4 metres along the plane:

work (in joules) = force (in newtons) × distance (in metres).
∴ work done = 250 × 4
= 1000 joules.

* Or by calculation, for in triangle *ABC*, *AB* = *BC* cos 60°. (See, 'Mathematics for Radiographers', p. 95.)

It is possible to tackle the problem another way, with instructive results, as follows. If a scale drawing is made (Fig. 19c) it is found that, in moving the body 4 metres up the plane it is raised *vertically* through a height of 2 metres.* Now, 500 newtons, the *whole* force of gravity on the body (and not merely a resolved part of it) acts vertically and the movement *in this direction* is 2 metres. Thus:

$$\text{work done} = 500 \times 2$$
$$= 1000 \text{ joules.}$$

This is the same answer as before. Hence in problems concerned with work we may either consider the distance moved and the component of the force *in this direction*, or the total force together with the distance moved *parallel to* the direction of this force (and independent of actual movement taking place).

EXAMPLE

Find the work done against gravity by a man weighing 60 kgm in climbing a mountain 1000 metres high.

As implied by the statement above, the amount of work done against gravity in such a case is independent of the route taken by the man. It is equal simply to the weight of the man (the force due to gravity) multiplied by the *vertical* distance climbed (i.e. parallel to the force).

$$\text{Work done} = \text{force (in newtons)} \times \text{distance (in metres).}$$
$$= (60 \times 9 \cdot 81) \times 1000$$
$$= 588{,}600 \text{ joules.}$$

EXERCISES

1. When does a force do work? What are the joule and the erg? How may the amount of work done by a force be found,
   (a) when movement is entirely in the direction of the force,
   (b) when the force supplied and the resulting movements are *not* in the same direction?

2. Find the work done against gravity by a man weighing 70 kgm when he climbs 5 metres up a flight of stairs?

3. An object weighing 4 gm is pushed 7 cm up a slope which makes an angle of 25° with the horizontal. If friction can be neglected, how much work (in ergs) is done? (You may use trigonometry or a scale drawing.)

4. The tube head of an X-ray set weighs 150 kgm. What work is done in raising it 100 cm?

---

* Again, in triangle XYZ, $XY = YZ \cos 60°$.

4

ENERGY

The word *energy* is used in Physics to denote much the same thing as it denotes in everyday parlance. An energetic person—a person with a great deal of energy—is one who can do a great deal of work. In Physics, the amount of energy possessed by a body is a measure of the amount of *work* it can do, using the term *work* in the sense in which it was defined above (p. 39).

Potential Energy

There are various ways in which energy—the ability to do work— may be given to a body. A grandfather clock weight, when raised, can, as it descends, drive the clock and so do *work* for us. In fact, we have given *energy* to the weight in raising it, and this energy, which has been stored by the weight, is called *potential* energy. Potential energy is to be associated with some special position or shape given to a body. A coiled-up clock spring, a compressed (or extended) spiral spring, a piece of stretched rubber, a quantity of compressed gas, and a quantity of liquid pumped from a lower level to a higher level, are all instances of the storing up of potential energy, for in each case work can be done by the body or quantity of matter in returning to its former shape or position. We shall meet other important examples of potential energy in our study of magnetism and electricity. It is very important to realize that the amount of work done *by* a body in giving up its energy is merely equal to the amount of work which had to be done *on* it to impart the energy to it. For instance, the work done by the clock weight in descending is exactly equal to the work which had to be done to raise it. Since energy is a measure of the amount of work which a body can do, the same units (i.e. units of work) are employed for it.

EXAMPLES

1. An object of mass 15 kgm is raised vertically through 3 m. What is its increase in potential energy (in joules)?

   As stated above, the change in potential energy will be equal to the work done in raising body against the force of gravity.

   $$\text{Force (in newtons)} = \text{mass (in kgm)} \times \text{acceleration (in m per sec}^2)$$
   $$= 15 \times 9 \cdot 81 = 147 \cdot 2 \text{ newtons.}$$
   $$\text{Work done} = \text{force (in newtons)} \times \text{distance moved (in metres)}$$
   $$= 147 \cdot 2 \times 3 = 442 \text{ joules.}$$

2. An object of mass 2 gm descends 3 cm vertically. How much potential energy (in ergs) has it lost?

$$\text{Force} = \text{mass (in gm)} \times \text{acceleration (in cm per sec}^2)$$
$$= 2 \times 981 = 1962 \text{ dynes.}$$
$$\text{Work done (in ergs)} = \text{force (in dynes)} \times \text{distance (in cm)}$$
$$= 1962 \times 3$$
$$= 5886 \text{ ergs.}$$

Kinetic Energy

In order to set a body in motion a force must be applied to it, and since this force produces a movement in its own direction, it *does work* in generating the motion. The work done in this way is 'stored up' in the motion itself as *energy* of motion, or *kinetic* energy as it is called. In coming to rest again the body loses its kinetic energy, and in so doing it does an amount of work exactly equal to the amount which had to be done on it to generate the motion. For example, when the brakes of a moving vehicle are applied to bring it to a standstill, the kinetic energy of the vehicle is used up in doing work against the resistance offered by the force of friction on the brake drums, and the amount of work done in this way is equal to the work which had to be done to generate the vehicle's motion in the first place.

The kinetic energy of a body will obviously depend on the *speed* at which it is going. It will also depend on the *mass* of the body, for more work has to be done to generate a given speed in a massive body than in a light one. It is an easy matter to find an expression for the kinetic energy of a body in terms of its mass and its velocity.

Denote its mass by m and its velocity by v. Then its kinetic energy will be equal to the amount of work necessary to give a body of mass m a velocity of v. This amount of work will be equal to the force p applied to the body to generate the motion, multiplied by the distance s over which it acts. But the force p acting on the body of mass m (initially at rest) produces an acceleration a, where

$$p = ma.$$

Also, from one of the equations of accelerated motion we have

$$v^2 = 2as,$$
$$\text{or} \qquad s = \frac{v^2}{2a}.$$

Then, kinetic energy = work done by force p over distance s

$$= p \cdot s$$
$$= ma \cdot \frac{v^2}{2a} \text{ (substituting for } p \text{ and } s\text{)}$$
$$= \tfrac{1}{2}mv^2.$$

It is extremely important to realize that since the value of p has been expressed in absolute units in order to make use of Newton's Second Law of Motion, the expression $\frac{1}{2} mv^2$ gives the kinetic energy of the body in *absolute* units of work. Thus, if the mass is in kilogrammes and the velocity is in metres per second, the kinetic energy is given in *joules*. For m in gm and v in cm per sec, the kinetic energy is given in *ergs*.

EXAMPLES

1. What is the kinetic energy (in joules) of a mass of 4 kgm after falling under gravity, through 3 m from rest?

    Now, $v^2 = u^2 + 2as$ (p. 29)

    $u = 0$ (from rest), $a = 9\cdot81$ m per sec^2 (for gravity), $s = 3$ m.

    $\therefore \qquad v^2 = 2 \times 9\cdot81 \times 3$

    Then, kinetic energy $= \frac{1}{2} m v^2$

    $\qquad\qquad\qquad = \frac{1}{2} \times 4 \times 2 \times 9\cdot81 \times 3$

    $\qquad\qquad\qquad = 117\cdot7$ joules.

2. An alpha particle (the nucleus of a helium atom) of mass $6\frac{2}{3} \times 10^{-24}$ gm is moving at a speed of 10^9 cm per sec. What is its kinetic energy in ergs? (See footnote p. 33.)

    Kinetic energy $= \frac{1}{2} mv^2$ (m in gm, v in cm per sec.)

    $\qquad\qquad = \frac{1}{2} \times 6\frac{2}{3} \times 10^{-24} \times (10^9)^2$

    $\qquad\qquad = \frac{1}{2} \times \frac{20}{3} \times 10^{-6}$

    $\qquad\qquad = 3\frac{1}{3} \times 10^{-6}$ ergs.

The Conservation of Energy

It is interesting to give simultaneous consideration to the potential and kinetic energies of a falling body. Suppose a body of mass m has fallen from rest through a distance h. Then the potential energy which it has lost is equal to the amount of work which would have to be done in *raising* it through this distance. This is equal to the distance h multiplied by the weight of the body.

If m is in kgm and h is in metres, the work done by the body in falling (that is the potential energy lost) will be mgh joules, where g is the acceleration due to gravity (in m per sec^2).

Now a body falling from rest through a distance h acquires a velocity of v given by

$$v^2 = 2gh \text{ (p. 30)}.$$

Therefore, the kinetic energy which it has gained $= \frac{1}{2} mv^2$
$$= \frac{1}{2} m(2gh)$$
$$= mgh.$$

But this is equal to the potential energy lost. It follows that the total mechanical energy (potential plus kinetic) of the body remains unchanged as it falls, for we have shown that at any point in the fall the potential energy which has been lost has been replaced by an exactly equivalent amount of kinetic energy. This is an example of one of the most fundamental principles of Physics, namely that energy can neither be created nor destroyed, but merely changed from one form into an exactly equivalent amount of another form.*

EXAMPLES

1. An object of mass 2 kgm is dropped over a cliff. Its velocity on reaching the ground is 50 m per sec. Through what height did it fall?
   Kinetic energy at end of fall (in joules)
$$= \frac{1}{2} \times \text{(mass in kgm)} \times \text{(velocity in m per sec)}^2$$
$$= \frac{1}{2} \times 2 \times 50^2 = 2500 \text{ joules}.$$
   Potential energy lost (in joules)
$$= \text{(mass in kgm)} \times \text{(acceleration due to gravity in m per sec}^2)$$
$$\times \text{(height in m)}$$
$$= 2 \times 9 \cdot 81 \times h.$$
   Now, kinetic energy gained = potential energy lost.
$$\therefore \qquad 2500 = 19 \cdot 62 \, h$$
   or, $\qquad h \quad = 127 \cdot 4$ metres.

2. A proton (the nucleus of a hydrogen atom) of mass $1\frac{2}{3} \times 10^{-24}$ gm 'falls' through an *electric* field (just as the mass in Ex. 1, p. 44, falls through the earth's *gravitational field*) and in doing so loses $0 \cdot 3 \times 10^{-6}$ ergs of potential energy. What velocity will it have acquired in consequence? (See footnote, p. 33.)
   From the Law of Conservation of Energy,
   $\qquad$ potential energy lost = kinetic energy gained.
   $\therefore$ kinetic energy gained $= 0 \cdot 3 \times 10^{-6}$
$$= 3 \times 10^{-7} \text{ ergs}.$$
$$\therefore \qquad \frac{1}{2}mv^2 = 3 \times 10^{-7},$$

* Einstein showed, however, that mass itself must be regarded as a form of energy, since a mass m gm of matter can be completely converted into mc^2 ergs of energy, where c is the velocity of light in cm per sec. Nuclear physics provides many examples of such transformations of mass to energy and *vice-versa*. (See, for instance, 'Radiation Physics in Radiology', pp. 41, 42.)

or $\qquad v^2 = \dfrac{2 \times 3 \times 10^{-7}}{m}$

$\qquad\qquad\quad = \dfrac{2 \times 3 \times 10^{-7}}{\frac{5}{3} \times 10^{-24}}$ (substituting for m)

$\qquad\qquad\quad = 36 \times 10^{16}.$

Whence, $\qquad v = 6 \times 10^8$ cm per sec.

Forms of Energy

Potential and kinetic energy are examples of *mechanical* energy. Energy can take other forms, however. We have seen that when the brakes of a moving vehicle are applied, the kinetic energy of the vehicle is used up in doing work against the forces of friction in the brakes. If the brakes were to be examined immediately after the vehicle had stopped they would be found to be *hot*. In fact *heat* has been generated, and is actually another form of energy into which the kinetic energy has been transformed. The fact that heat is another form of energy is more clearly demonstrated by the following example. Heat produced by the fire in a steam engine heats the water and generates steam. This steam is in a highly compressed state in the boiler, and in this condition it possesses potential energy, energy which has ultimately been derived from the heat of the fire. Inside the cylinder of the engine this potential energy of the steam is converted into kinetic energy as the steam expands, and the kinetic energy of the moving parts of the engine may be utilized to do work, such as raising a weight, or pumping water from a lower level to a higher level. Thus it is seen that as a result of a chain of energy transformations heat has ultimately done work for us. Put another way, heat can impart the capability of doing work, and must therefore be a form of energy.

Sound and light can also be shown to be forms of energy. It is fairly easy to see this in the case of the former. For example, it is well known that the sounding of a particular note of an instrument will cause a string tuned to the same note on another instrument in the vicinity to vibrate, a phenomenon known as *resonance*. In setting the second string in motion the sound must exert a force on it, producing movement against resistance. In other words work can be done by sound, and it must therefore be a form of *energy*.

We shall see in our study of electricity that an electric current acts as a conveyor of energy from one part of an electric circuit to another. Thus, when an electric current is passed through a filament of an electric lamp, energy conveyed to the lamp by the current is converted into heat and light energy.

In all energy transformations it is of the utmost importance to remember that the total amount of energy is neither increased nor decreased, for where one form of energy is converted simultaneously into a number of different forms, the sum total of the various forms into which it has been converted is always equal to the initial energy.

POWER

The more powerful an engine is, the more work it can do in a given time. Thus *power* is measured by the *rate* at which work is done, the units being joules (or ergs) per second. James Watt introduced as a *unit* of power the rate at which he considered an average cart horse would work. This unit, which he called one *horse power*, corresponds to 746 joules per second, and is, in fact, a rather optimistic estimate of a horse's ability!

EXAMPLE

A certain engine is able to raise a load of 1000 kgm vertically through 6 m in 30 sec. What is the power of the engine?

$$\text{The work done} = 1000 \times 9.81 \times 6$$
$$= 58,860 \text{ joules.}$$
$$\text{Hence, the rate of doing work} = \frac{58,860}{30}$$
$$= 1962 \text{ joules per sec}$$
$$= \frac{1962}{746} = 2.6 \text{ horse power.}$$

EXERCISES

1. What does 'power' measure? Name and define the units of power.
2. A man weighing 70 kgm runs up a flight of stairs, a height of 10 m, in 6 sec. At what horse power does he work? Comment on this answer.
3. An X-ray tube head of mass 150 kgm has to be raised through a height of one metre in 30 sec. What power is required?

MACHINES

In everyday language a 'machine' usually signifies a more or less complicated mechanism designed to carry out some special operation. Thus a sewing machine automatically *stitches* for us, and a printing machine automatically *prints* for us. The latter may even cut from a long roll the pieces of paper as they are printed, and fold and count them afterwards.

In Physics, on the other hand, the word *machine* is used to denote *any* piece of apparatus, however simple, which enables us to overcome a given resistance, or deal with a given load, *more effectively*. It usually (though not always) makes it possible for the force (which may be called the *effort*) applied to the machine to be appreciably smaller than the *load* dealt with; or else it makes it possible to apply the effort in a more convenient manner than would be possible without the 'machine'.

The Lever

This is perhaps the simplest of all machines, in the sense in which we are using the word. We may consider it to consist merely of a straight rod, pivoted at a certain point along its length. A common example is that of the *crowbar* (Fig. 20).

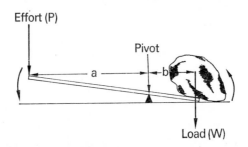

Fig. 20. The crowbar.

A stout bar is placed with one end under the object to be raised (the 'load' *W*) and, under the bar, near the same end of the rod, is placed the 'pivot' or 'fulcrum', being any small hard object (such as a block of wood) on which the bar can rest. The 'effort' *P*—the force which is to deal with the 'load'—is applied at the other end of the bar.

When the effort (exerted *downwards*) is just sufficient to raise the load, it follows from what has been said about moments (p. 16) that:

moment of effort about pivot = moment of load about pivot,

$$\text{i.e.} \quad P \times a = W \times b,$$

$$\text{or} \quad \frac{W}{P} = \frac{a}{b}.$$

$$\text{In words,} \quad \frac{\text{load}}{\text{effort}} = \frac{\text{effort's arm}}{\text{load's arm}}.$$

Thus, if the effort's arm is 10 times the load's arm, the load can be 10 times the effort. The ratio load/effort is called the *mechanical advantage* of the machine.

By means of a crowbar having a mechanical advantage of 10, a man capable of exerting a force of 50 kgm wt could deal with a load of 500 kgm wt. Note, however, that as the load's arm is only one tenth of the effort's arm, the load will only move through one tenth of the corresponding distance moved by the effort. Thus, if the man moves his end of the crowbar down 30 cm, the load will only rise 3 cm.

The work done will, in each case, be given by the product of the force and the distance moved. Thus:

Work done *by* effort = $50 \times 9{\cdot}81 \times 0{\cdot}3 = 147{\cdot}15$ joules.
Work done *on* load = $500 \times 9{\cdot}81 \times 0{\cdot}03 = 147{\cdot}15$ joules.

That is, the work done *by* the effort exactly equals the work done *on* the load. This is true only if the machine can be so well made that no work is wasted, for instance in overcoming friction. Otherwise more work would have to be done by the effort to do the same amount of work on the load. The ratio of the work *got out* of the machine to the corresponding work which must be *put in* therefore has a value of *unity* only if the machine is perfect; in general it will be *less* than unity. In fact this ratio is a measure of the *efficiency* of the machine and is usually expressed as a *percentage*.

The Windlass

A simple machine which finds wide application is known as a windlass (Fig. 21).

A force, F, is applied to the handle of the crank in such a way as to always act at right-angles to the arm of the crank. Then as the crank is turned the cord winds round the drum and the weight, W, (attached to the free end of the cord) is raised. In one revolution the load will rise

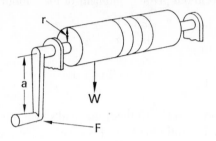

Fig. 21. The windlass.

through a distance equal to the circumference of the drum ($2\pi r$). Correspondingly the effort will act over a distance equal to $2\pi a$.

Therefore, if the machine is perfect, we may write:

$$\frac{\text{load}}{\text{effort}} \quad \frac{\text{distance moved by effort}}{\text{distance moved by load}}$$

$$= \frac{2\pi a}{2\pi r} = \frac{a}{r}.$$

For example, if the crank has a length five times that of the radius of the drum, an effort of only one fifth of the load will be required.

Gears and Belted Pulleys

In a similar way it may be shown that two gear wheels engaging with each other (or two pulley wheels carrying a belt), one of radius r and the other of radius R (Fig. 22), provide a mechanical advantage of R/r if there is no appreciable friction.

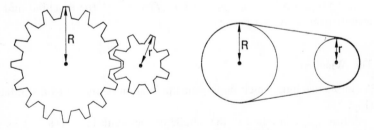

Fig. 22. Gears and pulley systems.

The Screw

Apart from its obvious use in holding parts of a structure together, the screw is also employed in numerous mechanisms, and in our sense of the word, it may be regarded as a *machine*. To elucidate this point, we

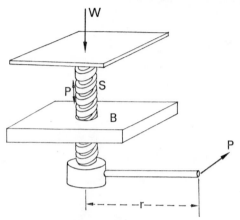

Fig. 23. The screw.

may consider the very simple (and not very practical!) arrangement shown in Fig. 23. Here a stout screw *S*, threaded through a fixed bush *B*, carries a load *W* at the top, and a crank arm (of radius *r*) at the bottom. The *pitch* of the screw is *p*, which means simply that for each revolution of the screw the load *W* is raised (or lowered) a distance *p*.

Suppose an effort *P* is applied in the usual way to the handle of the crank. Then, if the screw is of 100% efficiency:

$$\frac{\text{work done by effort}}{\text{in one revolution}} = \frac{\text{work done on load}}{\text{in one revolution}}$$

$$\therefore \quad P \times 2\pi r = W \times p,$$

or mechanical advantage $\dfrac{W}{P} = \dfrac{2\pi r}{p}$.

Thus a screw with a pitch of 1/10 in. and an arm of length 7 in. would have a mechanical advantage of

$$\frac{2 \times \pi \times 7}{1/10} \text{ or } 440.$$

The screw in a variety of practical forms is therefore a very useful mechanism to employ where large mechanical advantages are required. For example, where heavy loads are to be raised through relatively small distances some kind of *screw jack* is employed, and the same principle is often employed in an X-ray gantry for the purpose of raising and lowering the heavy tubehead.

CHAPTER 4
Heat

MEASUREMENT OF TEMPERATURE

Heat and Temperature

A distinction must first be made between the meanings of the words
heat and temperature—which in everyday language are often used as
though they were synonymous. It has already been seen that heat is, in
fact, a form of energy. It is not easy to express in words simply—and
at the same time precisely—the meaning of the *temperature* of a body,
except to say that it is a measure of its 'hotness'.

When a body gains heat, generally speaking (although not invariably,
see p. 68), a rise in temperature is produced. This is usually accompanied
by expansion, or in the case of a quantity of gas prevented from ex-
panding, by a rise in pressure. There may also be changes in the physical
and electrical properties of a substance. Thus there may be a change of
state, as when ice melts into water, whilst (in general) the electrical
resistance of a metal increases with rise of temperature.

Thermometers

Changes in any of these properties (volume, length, electrical resistance
(see p. 130), etc.) may be employed to assess the corresponding changes
in temperature which they accompany. Instruments for this purpose
are known as thermometers, and by far the majority of them make use
of expansion, usually of a liquid, although some types employ the
expansion of a solid or even of a gas. The commonest form of thermometer is shown diagrammatically in Fig. 24, and consists of a thin-walled
glass bulb *A* at the end of a capillary tube *B*. The bulb is filled with the
liquid (usually *mercury* or coloured *alcohol*) which extends into the
capillary tube. Marked on the latter is a scale *C*. As the liquid in the
bulb expands, the level of the liquid in the tube rises. Once the level is

steady, the corresponding reading on the scale is an indication of the
temperature, in the units represented by the scale divisions.

The clinical thermometer, used for measurement of body temperature,
is of special interest. Such thermometers are required to be accurate
and easily read, but are used over only a very limited temperature
range. Also it would obviously be inconvenient to have to read the
thermometer whilst it was in the patient's mouth, so it is necessary
that after removal from the patient the thermometer should still

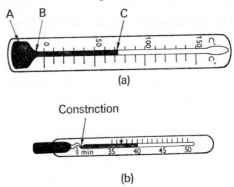

(a)

Constriction

(b)

Fig. 24a. A *mercury-in-glass* thermometer.

Fig. 24b. A *clinical* thermometer.

indicate the maximum temperature attained during the measurement
(the fall in recorded temperature must not at any rate exceed 0·2° F).
To this end a special construction is adopted as shown in Fig. 24b.
The mercury is normally all within the bulb, and does not expand
into the short stem until the temperature is within the limited range
of the calibration from 35–40° C (or 95–105° F, see p. 55). The scale
markings are then quite widely spaced so that it is possible to read to
1/10°, and to assist this reading the front face of the glass is curved to
form a cylindrical lens which provides a magnified image of the mercury
column. Now the capillary tube between the bulb and the calibrated
stem has a very narrow constriction, and, as the temperature rises, the
mercury is forced past this constriction owing to the very great forces
set up in expansion (see p. 57). On cooling (after removal from the
patient) the weight of the mercury column is insufficient, however, to
force its return past the constriction, and the mercury remains in the
stem to indicate the maximum temperature attained. After the reading
has been noted the mercury is shaken back into the bulb. It is importan

that a clinical thermometer should be accurate, and it is advisable to use one which has been checked against standards provided by one of the national standardizing laboratories (e.g. the National Physical Laboratory in Britain) thus ensuring that the reading is correct within 0·2° F.

Scales of Temperature

There are two scales of temperature in common use—the *Fahrenheit* scale and the *Celsius* (formerly *Centrigrade*) scale. On the Fahrenheit scale the freezing point of water is 32 degrees (32°) and the boiling point 212°, giving 180 Fahrenheit degrees between freezing point and boiling point. On the Celsius scale the freezing point is 0° and the boiling point 100°. Thus 100 Celsius degrees cover the same range as 180 Fahrenheit degrees, and it follows that the Celsius degrees are 'larger', 1 Celsius degree being equivalent to 180/100, or 9/5 Fahrenheit degrees.

In scientific work the Celsius scale is generally used, or a modification of this known as the *Absolute* scale (or sometimes *Kelvin* scale, after Lord Kelvin). Theoretically it appears that there is a lower limit to temperature (corresponding to the final cessation of the thermal movement of the molecules of matter, see p. 2) at about −273° C. This temperature is therefore taken as zero on the Absolute scale whilst still using the Celsius divisions or degrees. Thus a temperature on the Absolute scale (°A) is given with sufficient accuracy by adding 273° to the temperature on the Celsius scale.

Such calculations as the correction of dosemeter readings require a knowledge of room temperature in degrees Absolute, yet room thermometers commonly give the Fahrenheit temperature. Thus it is necessary to be able to convert temperatures on the Fahrenheit scale to Celsius and Absolute temperatures.

EXAMPLES

1. Room temperature is 77° F. Express this in degrees on the Absolute scale.
   77° F. corresponds to (77 − 32) or 45 Fahrenheit degrees above the freezing point of water.
   Now, as pointed out above, each Celsius degree corresponds to 9/5 Fahrenheit degrees.

   $$\therefore \ 45 \text{ Fahrenheit degrees} = 45 \times \frac{5}{9} \text{ Celsius degrees}$$

   $$= 25 \text{ Celsius degrees above the freezing point of water.}$$

As, on the Celsius scale, the freezing point of water is 0°, this temperature is in fact 25° C.

Thus the temperature on the Absolute scale is given by

$$(25 + 273) = 298° \text{ A.}$$

2. Express 10° C on the Fahrenheit scale.

10° C means 10 Celsius degrees above the freezing point of water, and each Celsius degree is equal to 9/5 Fahrenheit degrees.

$$\text{Therefore, } 10° \text{ C} \equiv \left(10 \times \frac{9}{5} \right)$$

= 18 degrees on the Fahrenheit scale above the freezing point of water (32° F)

$$\therefore 10° \text{ C} \equiv (18 + 32)° \text{ F}$$
$$= 50° \text{ F.}$$

EXERCISES

1. Express 72° F on the Absolute scale.
2. Express 17·5° C on the Fahrenheit scale.
3. Express 98·4° F on the Celsius scale.

THERMAL EXPANSION

Expansion of Solids

When a solid expands it retains its shape, that is, each linear dimension will increase in the same proportion. The amount of expansion is in general small, and it is difficult to observe the change except by using a system of levers or some similar device to magnify the increase in length. However, the fact that expansion does in fact occur may be demonstrated quite simply. For instance, a metal ball, which at room temperature will just pass through a ring, is unable to do so when heated, because of the resultant expansion.

The amount of expansion produced by a given temperature change varies with the material. This is represented by the *coefficient of linear expansion*, which is the increase in length per unit of original length (i.e. increase in length/original length) produced by a temperature rise of 1° C. Values of this coefficient are given in Table I (p. 63) for some materials of interest including Invar, a special nickel-iron alloy with a very small expansion, which finds considerable application in the construction of scientific apparatus.

The difference in expansion of differing materials can be demonstrated by heating a 'compound bar', consisting of two strips, one of brass and one of iron riveted together at a number of points along their lengths (Fig. 25). As the temperature rises the brass strip expands more than the iron, distorting the bar into a curve as shown in Fig. 25b. Quite thick compound bars can be made to bend in this manner, showing the great force exerted during expansion. It is the *magnitude* of this force which is often of such practical importance, even though the amount of expansion may be small.

A few applications, and X-ray tube design problems concerned with thermal expansion, will now be considered.

The compound bar described above is used as the basis of both a *thermostat* and a so-called *thermal delay-switch*. In the former case the current to the heating coil of, for instance, an oven or incubator passes along the bar and across a pair of contacts (*ab* in Fig. 25a) held together

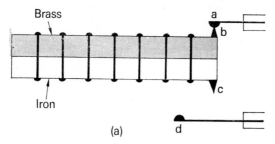

(a)

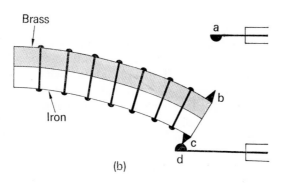

(b)

Fig. 25. Diagramatic representation of a compound bar thermal switch: (a) cold, (b) hot.

by a spring. As the bar in the oven becomes heated it bends until at a certain temperature (which is adjustable) the contacts are no longer made (Fig. 25b), and the heater current is cut off. As the bar (and oven) cools, it straightens and the contacts are remade, so that the heater current is switched on again. Thus the temperature of the oven is maintained within quite narrow limits as a result of the heater being switched on and off automatically at intervals. If the bar is heated by current flowing in a coil wrapped round the bar itself, the device becomes a thermal delay switch. Contacts *ab* are broken (Fig. 25b) at some definite time interval after switching on the heater current, as the temperature of the bar rises and it bends. Alternatively, contacts such as *cd* may be fitted, which are only *made* on completion of a certain interval after the start of the heater current. Such a device is sometimes used to prevent the high voltage being connected to a valve until the filament has had time to heat up to its operating temperature.

The following is an example of a problem created by differences in thermal expansion. The 'target' of an X-ray tube usually consists of a button of tungsten which is let into a large block of copper. The region round the focal spot becomes heated during use, and, in order that the heat shall be conducted away efficiently from the tungsten to the copper, the contact (or weld) between the two metals must be very close. However, these two metals now constitute a form of compound bar. They have very different coefficients of expansion (see Table I), and therefore very large forces are set up which will tend to break the weld and so damage the target. The tube designers consequently have to attach the tungsten in a manner which allows for movement relative to the copper during expansion, but maintains a reasonably good thermal contact between the materials.

If a bearing of a rotating spindle becomes too hot as the result of expansion of the spindle, it may become too tight and thus 'seize up'. The heating may be due to friction as a result of imperfect lubrication, or it may be due to heat conducted along the spindle, as for instance in a rotating anode type of X-ray tube where, of course, the anode itself becomes very hot. In order to avoid seizing, the bearing is in this case made a loose fit to allow for expansion, whilst at the same time measures are taken to reduce the rise in temperature of the spindle (see p. 72).

In many electrical devices, including valves and X-ray tubes, it is necessary to seal connecting wires into the wall of a glass bulb which has to be highly evacuated. If the seal then becomes heated, as will be the case for instance with the filament leads or anode connection of an X-ray tube, the metal and glass will expand. If the amounts of these expansions are not the same the forces set up may break the seal and so destroy the vacuum within the tube. Most metals expand more than glass (see Table I, p. 63), but as platinum and tungsten have similar coefficients of expansion to that of ordinary glass these materials were formerly used for such seals. Now special alloys, much cheaper than platinum, are available for this purpose, and their expansion may be chosen to match the particular type of glass used (usually boro-silicate glass, see Table I).

Expansion of Liquids

In the case of liquids (which have no fixed shape) we have only volume expansion to consider. The *coefficient of volume expansion* (the increase in volume per unit original volume for 1° C temperature rise) is listed in Table I for a number of liquids of particular interest. It will be seen that these coefficients are much greater than the values for solids (which are approximately three times the corresponding coefficients of linear expansion)—hence the general application of the expansion of liquids in thermometry.

As an X-ray set is operated, the oil which surrounds the tube (for insulation purposes) becomes heated and expands. In some designs (e.g. in superficial and diagnostic sets) this is allowed for by providing a set of bellows which can extend as the oil expands and so increase the effective volume of the tube housing containing the oil. The amount of expansion of the bellows is then a measure of the temperature rise in the oil, and a 'micro-switch' can be included so that the set is switched off at some level of expansion corresponding to the maximum oil temperature which can be permitted, thus avoiding overheating of the oil and tube. In other designs (e.g. in deep therapy sets) the tube housing is connected by pipes to a further tank into which the oil can expand.

It is commonly said that 'heat rises', and the phenomenon thus alluded to is also due to thermal expansion. If heat is applied locally to a quantity of liquid, the heated part expands and therefore becomes less dense than the surrounding liquid. The resultant force of buoyancy which is set up causes this liquid to rise through the denser parts, carrying with it the heat energy imparted to it. Cooler liquid flows in to take its place and in turn becomes heated and rises. Thus a stream of liquid, known as a *convection current*, circulates, carrying heat energy along with it. Convection currents as a means of heat transfer are considered further on p. 72.

A simple demonstration of convection currents is shown in Fig. 26. Some water is heated in a glass beaker by means of a small Bunsen flame; a few crystals of potassium permanganate (which are deep red) are dropped into the water above the heated spot. The crystals sink to the bottom and dissolve in the water to produce coloured streaks, which show a current of water rising to the surface from the heated spot. At the surface a great deal of the heat is lost, and the cooled liquid falls to the bottom again (down the sides of the beaker) to become heated once more. In this way a continuous circulation of water is set up.

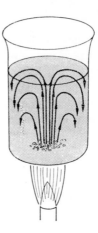

Fig. 26.

Expansion of Gases

Both the shape and volume of gases are determined by the vessel in which they are contained. If the volume is held constant, an *increase of pressure* takes the place of an increase of volume as the temperature rises. This pressure increase is associated with the increased bombardment of the walls of the vessel due to the increased velocity of the gas molecules with temperature. If, however, the gas is contained in a cylinder closed by a moveable piston, the gas can *increase its volume* and expand at constant pressure. The relationships between pressure (or volume) and temperature under these conditions can be stated thus—when a gas is heated at *constant volume* its pressure is proportional to the Absolute temperature ($p \propto T$, V constant); and *Charles' Law*—when a gas is heated at *constant pressure* its volume is proportional to the Absolute temperature ($V \propto T$, p constant).

EXAMPLE

The temperature of 120 cc of gas is raised from 6° C to 99° C, keeping the volume constant. If the initial pressure was 75 cm of mercury, calculate the pressure at the higher temperature. The gas is then heated further, allowing it to expand at constant pressure to a volume of 150 cc. Calculate the further rise in temperature.

$$\text{Initial temperature} = 6° \text{ C}$$
$$\equiv (6 + 273)° \text{ A}$$
$$= 279° \text{ A.}$$
$$\text{Similarly, final temperature} = 372° \text{ A.}$$

∴ at constant volume

$$\frac{\text{initial pressure}}{\text{final pressure}} = \frac{\text{initial Absolute temperature}}{\text{final Absolute temperature}},$$

or

$$\frac{75}{p} = \frac{279}{372},$$

whence, pressure $p = 100$ cm of mercury.

Then again, at constant pressure,

$$\frac{\text{initial volume}}{\text{final volume}} = \frac{\text{initial Absolute temperature}}{\text{final Absolute temperature}},$$

so

$$\frac{120}{150} = \frac{372}{T},$$

whence, $T = 465°$ A or 192° C.

That is, rise in temperature = 93 deg. on Celsius scale.

EXERCISES

1. A certain volume of gas is heated at constant volume from a temperature of 0° C to 91° C. The final pressure is 100 cm of mercury. Calculate the initial pressure.
2. Gas in a cylinder, initially at 19° C, is heated so that it expands at constant pressure from a volume of 40 cc to 50 cc. Calculate the temperature rise in degrees Celsius.

In correcting the reading of an X-ray exposure meter for variations in room temperature (cf. p. 4) we are concerned with the variation in the *mass* of gas in a given volume at constant pressure. This relationship may be obtained by application of the above laws. Thus if a mass (M_1 grammes) of gas is contained in a volume V_1 cc at a temperature of $T_1°$ A, then it follows that at the same pressure but at say, a higher temperature $T_2°$ A, the same mass M_1 of gas will be contained in a volume V_2 cc, where

$$\frac{V_2}{V_1} = \frac{T_2}{T_1},$$

whence, $\qquad V_2 = \frac{T_2}{T_1} V_1.$

Therefore the original volume V_1 will now contain a proportionately smaller mass of gas M_2, where

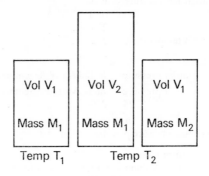

Fig. 27.

$$M_2 = \frac{V_1}{V_2} M_1 \text{ (see Fig. 27)}.$$

Whence, substituting for V_2, we get

$$M_2 = \frac{V_1}{\left(\dfrac{T_2}{T_1} \cdot V_1\right)} M_1,$$

or $\qquad \dfrac{M_2}{M_1} = \dfrac{T_1}{T_2}.$

In words, *the mass of gas contained in a given volume is inversely proportional to the absolute temperature, provided the pressure remains constant.*

It is implied above that as a gas is heated at constant pressure the volume of a given mass increases, or in other words its density decreases. This hot gas, therefore, will be lighter than the surrounding cooler gas, and will rise through it, carrying its heat with it. That is, *convection currents* are set up in the gas in exactly the same way as has been described for liquids (p. 59).

It is of interest to consider the expansion of gases in greater detail. Consider a volume of gas at 0° C and assume that it is heated through 1° C under constant pressure conditions. Then from the law stated above:

$$\frac{\text{final volume}}{\text{original volume}} = \frac{\text{final Absolute temperature}}{\text{original Absolute temperature}}$$

$$= \frac{274}{273}.$$

That is to say, for this 1° C temperature rise the volume increases by 1/273 of the original volume, which figure then corresponds to the coefficient of volume expansion as previously defined for solids and

TABLE I

	Solids		Liquids	
	Coefficient of Linear Expansion per °C	Coefficient of Volume Expansion per °C		Coefficient of Volume Expansion per °C
Aluminium	26×10^{-6}	0.78×10^{-4}	Alcohol	11×10^{-4}
Copper	17×10^{-6}	0.51×10^{-4}	Mercury	18×10^{-4}
Iron	12×10^{-6}	0.36×10^{-4}	Transformer	
Platinum	9×10^{-6}	0.27×10^{-4}	Oil	8×10^{-4}
Alloy for glass metal seal	5×10^{-6}	0.15×10^{-4}	Water (at 20° C)	2×10^{-4}
Boro-silicate glass	4.6×10^{-6}	0.14×10^{-4}		
Tungsten	4×10^{-6}	0.12×10^{-4}		
Invar	1×10^{-6}	0.03×10^{-4}		

liquids (p. 59). However, in this case the figure will vary with the temperature of the gas, being by similar reasoning 1/283 for a temperature rise from 10° C to 11° C, and so on. Nevertheless, by comparing such figures (1/273, or 3.66×10^{-3}) with the coefficients of volume expansion listed in Table I, it is seen that the expansion obtained with a gas at constant pressure is considerably greater than that for solids or liquids. It should also be noted here that, so long as this law of increase of volume at constant pressure applies, the coefficients of expansion calculated above apply to *any* gas.

Either the change of pressure of a gas at constant volume or the change of volume at constant pressure may be used to measure temperature. From what has been said immediately above, it is obvious that such thermometers are very 'sensitive', but they are not very convenient for general use.

There is sometimes a demonstration in an X-ray set of the fact that the expansion of gas is greater than for liquids. In the previous section it was explained that in some designs the expansion of the oil round the X-ray tube extends a set of bellows and operates, at some predetermined temperature, a safety switch which prevents further exposures until the tube has cooled. If however, because of a leak in the system, air should get into the oil, its expansion will be much greater than that of the oil it is replacing, so that the bellows are compressed and the safety switch operated at a much lower temperature than usual. The set is then switched off although it is not, in fact, overheated.

MEASUREMENT OF QUANTITY OF HEAT

If some hot liquid is placed into a cold vessel the liquid gets colder and the vessel hotter until they both reach the same temperature; that is, heat is transferred from the liquid to the vessel so long as a temperature difference exists. In dealing with such problems of heat transfer a unit of quantity of heat is required. In the Metric system this unit is the amount of heat required to raise the temperature of one gramme of water through 1° C and is called the *calorie* (cal).

EXAMPLE

Calculate the amount of heat (in calories) to raise the temperature of 35 gm water through 20 degrees Celsius.

To raise the temperature of 1 gm water though 1° C we require 1 calorie.

∴ to raise the temperature of 35 gm water through 1° C we require 35 calories.

∴ to raise the temperature of 35 gm water through 20° C we require (35 × 20) or 700 calories.

EXERCISES

1. Calculate the rise in temperature (in Celsius degrees) produced in 1½ litres of water by 2500 calories (1 cc of water weighs 1 gm).

The Mechanical Equivalent of Heat

It has already been pointed out (p. 46) that the heat is a form of energy, and therefore the units of energy (or work) can be used to measure quantity of heat. It was, in fact, careful experiments by Joule and others—showing a constant relationship between the amount of mechanical work done and the amount of heat produced (e.g. by friction) —which first established the principle of conservation of energy in these various forms. It is found that 4·18 joules of work (4·18 × 10⁷ ergs) correspond to one calorie, and this value (4·18 joules per cal) is known as the *mechanical equivalent of heat*. In fact, in scientific work, it is now customary to state the quantity of heat directly in *joules* instead of using the calorie for this purpose.

Specific Heat and Thermal Capacity; Calorimetry

If temperature change depends only on the amount of heat added or subtracted, then, for example, when a piece of copper weighing 100 gm and heated to 100° C is added to 100 gm water at 0° C we should expect the final temperature of the mixture to be 50° C, since the heat gained by the water is merely the heat lost by the copper. Actually, experiment shows it to be about 9° C, so that the amount of heat lost by the copper in cooling 91° raises the temperature of the same mass of water by only 9° (about a tenth of the temperature change in the copper). This variation in the temperature change for a given amount of heat added or subtracted, is expressed by the *specific heat* of a substance, which is defined as the amount of heat (in calories) which will raise the temperature of one gramme of the substance by 1° C. As one calorie is *defined* as the amount of heat to raise the temperature of one gramme of water by 1° C, the specific heat of water is unity. Also, it follows from the definition that the specific heat of any other substance is numerically equal to the ratio of the amount of heat to produce a certain temperature rise in a given mass of the substance, to that required to produce the same temperature rise in the same mass of water.

It is useful to consider this relationship in another way. If the specific heat of a substance is s cal gm per deg. C, this means that s calories will raise the temperature of one gramme by 1° C. Therefore *one* calorie will produce a temperature rise in one gramme of the substance of $1/s$ °C, or in other words, the temperature rise produced in a given mass by a given quantity of heat is inversely proportional to the specific heat of the substance.

Table II (p. 68) gives values of the specific heat for a number of common substances. It should be noted that the specific heat of water is the highest of all.

It will now be obvious that the temperature rise produced in a body by a given amount of heat depends on both the mass of the body and on its specific heat, s. In fact the heat required to raise the temperature of the body by 1° C will be s calories for each gramme of substance, or a total of $(m \times s)$ calories. This quantity, the amount of heat (in calories) to raise the temperature of the whole body 1° C, is termed the *thermal capacity* of the body.

We can now consider some practical points in the design of X-ray equipment which are concerned with problems of thermal capacity.

The focal spot on the anode of an X-ray tube becomes heated during an exposure, and it is necessary to avoid too great a rise in the temperature of the whole anode as this could lead to damage of the metal-glass seal or, in the case of a rotating anode tube, to excessive expansion and consequent seizing of the bearing. For a given heat quantity generated during an X-ray exposure it is therefore desirable to make the thermal capacity of the anode as large as possible. As already mentioned, the 'target' is made of tungsten, and from Table II it will be seen that this material has a low specific heat. However, this tungsten button is mounted in a large cylinder of copper, which has a comparatively high specific heat, and the thermal capacity (mass × specific heat) of the whole anode is kept high.

X-ray therapy tubes are operated continuously during quite long exposures (15 to 20 minutes) and it is necessary to remove heat by circulating a cooling liquid through the anode. As seen in Table II, water has a high specific heat and is therefore a very useful liquid for such a cooling system. For a given temperature difference between the in-going and out-going coolant, water will carry away more heat than the same weight of any other liquid. However, as mains water is not a good electrical insulator it is not always possible to employ water in such an X-ray tube cooling system, and oil (with good insulating properties) must be used instead (see Example below).

A further application of the principles of calorimetry in radiology is to be found in the field of radiation dosimetry. The energy *absorbed* from beams of such radiations as X-rays, gamma rays and electrons (i.e. the absorbed *dose*) ultimately all appears as heat in the absorbing medium,* and so can be measured by the methods of calorimetry (i.e. heat measurement). One *rad*, the unit of absorbed dose, is defined as an energy absorption of 100 ergs per gramme of medium. If therefore an X-ray beam is absorbed in, say, a piece of lead, under conditions where heat loss from the specimen is eliminated (or very small and known accurately), measurement of the heat produced will provide a measure of the energy absorbed within the specimen; or if *all* the energy of the beam is absorbed within the piece of lead, the heat produced will be a measure of the total energy conveyed by the beam.

Although this calorimetric estimation of absorbed dose is not in general convenient, and the energy absorption is usually calculated from the measurement of an ionization current produced in a small air cavity, calorimetry remains the fundamental method, and is therefore of great importance. Recent advances in technique, and in particular in the measurement of very small temperature changes of the order of 10^{-3} or 10^{-4} °C, have enabled accurate calorimetric measurements to be made for comparison with the air ionization results.

EXAMPLE

An X-ray tube cooling system is able to pump 10 litres of coolant through the anode each minute. The heat exchange within the anode produces a temperature rise in the coolant of 12° C. Compare the heat removed per minute when using water, and oil of specific heat 0·5 cal per gm per deg. C and density 0·8 gm per cc.

Mass of water pumped through per minute = 10,000 gm.
Thermal capacity of this mass of water = (10,000 × 1·00) cal per deg. C.
∴ heat removed for 12° C rise in temperature = 10,000 × 12
= 120,000 cal per min.
Mass of oil pumped through per minute = 10,000 × 0·8
= 8000 gm.
Thermal capacity of this mass of oil = (8000 × 0·5) cal per deg. C
∴ heat removed for 12° C rise in temperature = 4000 × 12
= 48,000 cal per min.

i.e. water would remove 120,000/48,000, or about 2·5 times as much heat per minute as the oil.

* Provided that none of this energy is utilized in producing permanent changes in the absorbing medium such as are brought about by chemical changes or nuclear reactions.

TABLE II

Specific Heats in cal per gm per deg. C			
Beryllium	0·43	Water	1·00
Aluminium	0·22	Alcohol	0·58
Copper	0·09	Transformer oil	0·5
Iron	0·11	Glass	0·16
Lead	0·031	Rubber	0·40
Tungsten	0·034	Wood	~0·4
		Wax	~0·7

EXERCISES

1. Calculate the amount of heat (in calories and in joules) necessary to raise the temperature of a copper anode by 60 degrees Fahrenheit. The mass of the anode is 1400 gm and its specific heat 0·09 cal per gm per deg. C. (N.B. You must use a temperature rise in deg. C to obtain an answer in calories. Assume that 4·2 joules equals 1 calorie.)

CHANGE OF STATE; MELTING, VAPORIZATION AND BOILING

When a solid changes into a liquid or a liquid into a vapour (or *vice versa*) a *change of state* is said to occur. These changes from solid to liquid or liquid to vapour may be brought about by the addition of heat, and the reverse changes by the removal of heat. For example, ice may be turned into water by heating it, and so conversely water may be turned into ice by taking heat away from it by means of a refrigerator. Whilst these changes of state are taking place no change of temperature occurs, in spite of the fact that heat is being supplied or removed. When heat is utilized in this way to change the state of a substance it is termed *latent* heat, since its presence is not made evident by the usual change of temperature. The *latent heat* of a substance is then defined as the amount of heat (in calories) to change one gramme of the substance from one state to the other. Thus the latent heat of fusion of ice is 80 cal per gm and the latent heat of vaporization of water is 539 cal per gm (at 100° C).

Since heat is a form of energy, any change in the amount of heat possessed by a quantity of matter represents a change in its total energy. We have already observed (Chap. 1) that the molecules of a vapour are much further apart than the molecules of the corresponding liquid, whilst the liquid molecules are much further apart than the molecules of the solid from which it was formed. Thus we may conclude that the latent heat supplied to a solid in order to convert it to a liquid is responsible for the work which has to be done in separating the molecules of the solid, against the forces of attraction which hold them together (and in imparting kinetic energy to them). Similarly the latent heat supplied to a liquid, in order to convert it to a vapour, is required for the work which must be done in separating the molecules of the liquid still further (and in increasing still more their kinetic energy) to form the vapour.

Generally speaking, the volume of vapour formed as a liquid boils is very much greater than the volume of the liquid from which it is formed. Work has to be done against atmospheric pressure in bringing about this increase in volume, and it follows that any change in atmospheric pressure will involve a corresponding change in the amount of energy required to convert a given quantity of liquid into vapour. It is not surprising to find, therefore, that the temperature at which a liquid boils depends on this pressure, the higher the pressure the higher the boiling point, and *vice versa*. Thus water which boils at 100° C under an atmospheric pressure of 76 cm of mercury will boil at about 89° C when the pressure falls to 50 cm (corresponding to a height of some 3300 m above sea level), and at 0° C for a pressure of 0·46 cm. On the other hand it will not boil until 200° C is attained when under a pressure of sixteen atmospheres (corresponding to conditions in the boiler of a steam engine).

Some vapour does form above the surface of a liquid even at temperatures below the boiling point. If this vapour is removed, further vapour is formed and the liquid evaporates. Thus if there is a breeze removing the vapour from above a puddle of water it gradually evaporates and dries up, but if the water is in a sealed vessel a certain amount of vapour is formed to 'saturate' the space above the liquid, and no further evaporation takes place. The saturation pressure attained by the vapour increases with temperature until the liquid finally boils.

If the latent heat required to form the vapour is not supplied from outside, it must be taken from the liquid itself, thereby cooling it. Thus if, for instance, ether is spilled on the hand it feels cold, owing to the rapid evaporation which takes place.

To some extent direct evaporation to vapour also occurs over solids, and the amount of this which occurs again increases with temperature.

Thus the heated filament of a valve or X-ray tube continually loses some of its matter by evaporation, becomes thinner and finally breaks (after some 10 per cent loss of weight). This evaporation is greatly accelerated if the filament is run at a very high temperature (e.g. to provide very high tube current at low kV), with consequent shortening of the filament life.

METHODS OF TRANSFER OF HEAT

Conduction

If one end of a poker is pushed into a fire, the other end quickly becomes too hot to hold. Heat energy is obviously being transferred from one end to the other, and we say that the process is due to *conduction*. What do we mean by this, and how does it come about?

We have already had occasion to refer to the fact that when heat energy is added to a solid, the energy associated with the vibration of its atoms or molecules about their mean position is increased, a phenomenon manifested by a rise in temperature. Now, if one part only of a solid is heated the vibrational energy of the atoms or molecules directly affected is increased, and the temperature of the heated portion rises. By what we may crudely term a 'jostling' process some of this vibrational energy begins to be handed on to neighbouring atoms or molecules not directly affected by the heating process, and gradually the energy spreads to more and more remote parts of the solid. It is to this process that we give the name conduction.

In view of the mechanism of the process it is not surprising that substances differ in their conducting powers. Thus, in contrast to the metal poker, one end of a glass rod may be maintained at red heat whilst the other end is held in the hand with comfort. The metal of which the poker is made is said to have a higher *thermal conductivity* than glass. All metals are more or less good conductors of heat, being in general better in this respect than solid non-metals.

Liquids and gases are on the whole much poorer conductors than solids, although this fact is often masked by the presence of convection currents (see p. 59, 63) which greatly assist the transfer of heat.

The following simple experiment (Fig. 28) demonstrates the poor conductivity of water. A piece of ice is weighted so that it sinks to the bottom of a test tube nearly full of water. The upper part only of the test tube is heated, thereby avoiding convection currents which, by their nature, rise. It is found that the conductivity of the water is so low that the water in the upper part of the test tube can be brought to the boil without melting the ice at the bottom.

In general, gases are the poorest conductors of all, a fact which accounts for the heat-insulating (i.e. poorly conducting) properties of fibrous and porous materials such as cork, feathers, dry wood, woollen articles, etc. Apart from the fact that the actual materials of which these substances are made are poor conductors, they contain as part of their structure enormous numbers of small air spaces (each space being more or less isolated from its neighbours, thus preventing the transfer of heat by convection currents), the presence of which leads to a very low overall thermal conductivity.

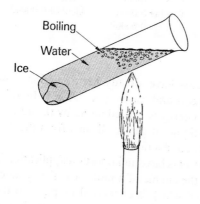

Fig. 28. Demonstration of poor conductivity of water.

The relative conducting powers of different substances may be compared by their *coefficients of thermal conductivity*. These coefficients are a measure of the rate at which the substance conducts heat under standard conditions, corresponding to the number of calories conducted per second between opposite faces of a unit cube when the temperature difference between the faces is 1° C.

Table III (p .72) gives thermal conductivities for a number of substances of interest.

It will be seen that the thermal conductivity of copper is comparatively high, and this is one of the reasons for the choice of copper in the construction of fixed anodes in X-ray tubes. The heat generated at the tungsten target is efficiently conducted away through the copper, and local overheating of the focal spot is avoided. In some designs of diagnostic rotating anode tubes the opposite procedure is adopted. Here, as has been pointed out already (p. 58) it is necessary to avoid overheating of the anode bearing. Thus, in order to minimize conduction of heat from the anode a section of low conductivity steel (see Table II) is inserted in the spindle between it and the bearing (see also p. 74).

TABLE III

Coefficients of Thermal Conductivity							
Metals		Solid Non-Metals		Liquids		Gases	
Copper	0·92	Wood (0·001— 0·003)		Water	0·0014	Air	0·00006
Tungsten	0·35	Glass	0·002	Transformer		Hydrogen	
Steel	0·12	Cork	0·0001	Oil	0·0004		0·00033
Lead	0·08	Rubber	0·0003	Alcohol	0·00042		
Silver	0·97	Felt	0·00009				

Convection

Convection currents have already been mentioned in connection with expansion of liquids and gases (pp. 59, 63). In this method of heat transfer the heat energy is carried along by the actual movement of the molecules of the liquid or gas, as distinct from the 'handing on' process which constitutes conduction.

Convection currents have an important application in cooling systems. For instance, in the engine of a motor car the cylinders are surrounded by a water 'jacket' which is connected by pipes to the top and bottom of the radiator. Convection currents are set up in the water round the hot cylinders, and the water flows from this jacket to the top of the radiator. Here it begins to cool, sinks to the bottom of the radiator through pipes fitted with cooling fins, and flows back again to the bottom of the water jacket. In this way heat is continuously carried away from the cylinders by the circulating water and the cylinder temperature is prevented from rising too high.

In some cars the flow of cooling liquid is increased by the use of a pump—the heat then being removed by 'forced convection' currents, and a similar arrangement may be employed to provide cooling for an X-ray tube anode.

Convection currents also represent the main method of heat transfer within the oil surrounding an X-ray tube, thus preventing overheating of parts of the tube and oil, and distributing the heat over the tube housing, whence it is lost by radiation and convection currents in the air. It is for this reason that it is usually recommended that if an X-ray tube is operated with the tube axis vertical, the anode should be at the *lower* position. The oil round the anode becomes heated and convection currents are set up, thus removing the heat and distributing it throughout the housing. If the anode is at the top, heat can pass through the oil by conduction only. Because liquids are relatively poor conductors the oil and the anode may become overheated, even with the tube operated under exposure conditions which are normally satisfactory. As a result, the target may suffer mechanical damage (e.g. melting), whilst the insulating properties of the oil may be permanently impaired.

Radiation

The radiation of heat energy—the third way in which heat may be transmitted from one place to another—does not depend on the presence of *any* material medium, solid, liquid, or gas. In the form of radiation, heat energy can be transmitted from one place to another through free space. That this is so is obvious from the fact that, for the majority of the distance, the heat from the sun travels through free space to the earth.

The nature of heat radiation cannot be discussed in any detail here (see also p. 217), but some of its properties and some of the phenomena associated with it are easily demonstrated.

For instance, we are all familiar with the fact that when a cloud moves across the sun, the direct heat from the sun is cut off *at once* by the cloud. This fact clearly demonstrates that heat radiation travels at great speed. Heat radiation shares this high speed with light and other forms of radiation such as wireless waves and X-rays, all of which have the same general nature (p. 223). Through free space the speed is actually about 3×10^8 m per second, so that heat and light radiation from the sun takes only about 8 minutes to do the journey.

It is also easy to demonstrate that heat radiation travels through a given substance (e.g. air) in straight lines. A small intense source of heat such as an arc lamp may be placed opposite, say, a triangular-shaped hole in a cardboard screen, a short distance behind which is a piece of heat-sensitive paper. The latter is impregnated with a chemical which changes colour when heated. It is found that a coloured area appears on the heat-sensitive paper, triangular in shape, whose position and size correspond to the area heated, on the assumption that the heat radiation travels in straight lines from the source.

Like some of its companion radiations, heat radiation can be reflected by suitable surfaces. Thus a polished metal surface is employed in an electric fire to concentrate the heat into a beam in the forward direction.

The rate of radiation of heat energy per unit area from a body depends on the nature of its surface. At the same temperature a dull black surface will emit more heat radiation per second than a polished metal or white surface. Thus a radiator will be more efficient if painted dull black, as the radiation loss will then be a maximum.

The rate of radiation also depends on the temperature of the body, being proportional to the fourth power of temperature on the Absolute scale. If a body is at the same temperature as its surroundings it is emitting heat radiation itself, but receiving back radiation at the same rate from its surroundings. If, however, it is at a higher temperature than its surroundings, the rate of emission of radiation from the body will exceed the rate at which it receives heat from the surroundings, and there will be a gradual loss of heat by the body. This rate of loss of heat will therefore be proportional to the difference of the fourth powers of the Absolute temperatures of the body and its surroundings. For small excesses this is approximately proportional to the actual difference between these temperatures, but increases rapidly for greater temperature differences.

This result means that heat loss by radiation becomes appreciable only at fairly high temperatures. Thus radiation of heat from a whole X-ray tube in its housing, only a few degrees above room temperature, is not an efficient process. In a diagnostic X-ray set with no forced cooling (such as is used in therapy sets), although the rate of heat dissipation may be high during the short exposures, it is this slow rate of radiation (and to some extent convection) loss which ultimately limits the rate at which exposures may be made on the set.

Another example of the application of radiation loss is found in some rotating anode tubes. It has already been mentioned that in some types a poor thermal conductor is inserted in the anode stem in order to reduce the heat transfer to the bearing. In this design the target must lose its heat efficiently by radiation to the rest of the X-ray tube. To this end the anode is in the form of a disc (large surface area) and made wholly of tungsten, which has a low specific heat and a high melting point, so that the temperature of the disc is allowed to become very high. A baffle plate is fitted between the anode and the rotating bearing to minimize heat radiation to this part of the tube.

EXERCISES

1. Explain the three methods by which heat may be transferred. Give examples of the application of these methods by X-ray tube designers.
2. Explain why a dull black body cools more quickly than one initially at the same temperature and of similar shape but which is highly polished. Why will both bodies finally reach the same temperature as their surroundings?

CHAPTER 5

Magnetism

MAGNETS; MAGNETIC POLES

The fact that electric and magnetic phenomena are closely related makes the study of magnetism an essential accompaniment to the study of electricity. The present chapter is concerned mainly with those magnetic phenomena which have a bearing on radiological physics (with special reference to measuring instruments and electrical supply circuits) and for this reason it lays no claim to being by any means exhaustive.

It was discovered in very early times—probably by the Chinese—that if a piece of lodestone (an iron ore which is naturally magnetized) was suspended by a fine thread it always came to rest lying in one particular direction. For this reason, probably in the first or second century A.D., it was applied in a crude fashion to navigation. No further study of magnetic phenomena seems to have been undertaken until the Middle Ages, notably by Peregrine (thirteenth century) and Gilbert (sixteenth century).

If a piece of lodestone is dropped into iron filings it is found that, although the filings cling to some extent to almost all parts of the lodestone's surface, they are more or less concentrated into two opposite regions—often near the extremities of the lodestone. The piece of lodestone behaves, in fact, as though its magnetism were concentrated into these two special regions which are known as the magnetic *poles* of the lodestone, and the lodestone itself can be termed a magnet. It is found that a small group of so-called *ferro-magnetic* materials, which includes iron, nickel, cobalt and many alloys of these elements, although normally not showing the natural magnetism of lodestone, can, in fact be magnetized, and nowadays such materials, magnetized with the aid of powerful electric currents, have completely replaced any use of lodestone.

The simplest form of artificial magnet is the *bar* magnet, which usually consists of a straight rectangular strip or cylindrical rod of magnetized steel. If a bar magnet is dipped into iron filings the two poles are shown to be roughly at the ends. Again, if such a magnet is suspended by means of a fine thread so that it can swing in a horizontal plane, it is found that, after being displaced from its rest position, it always settles in such a way that its axis lies in one particular (and approximately north-south) direction. For this reason the pole of the magnet which is situated at the end which always points northwards is called the *north-seeking pole* or simply the *north pole* of the magnet. The other pole is called the *south-seeking* or *south pole*.

Let us suppose that one bar magnet has been suspended in the manner described, and that a second one is also available. Then, if one end of the second magnet is brought near to one end of the first, it is found that, when these two poles are similar (or *like* poles as they are called), the pole belonging to the suspended magnet moves away from the other, showing that a force of repulsion exists between them. When the two poles concerned are *unlike*—a north and a south pole—a force of attraction between them can be shown to exist in a similar manner.

This demonstrates the truth of what is often referred to as the First Law of Magnetism: 'like poles repel, unlike poles attract each other.' It should be realized from Newton's Third Law of Motion (p. 34) that this force of attraction or repulsion is a *mutual* one.

The fact that one magnet is able to influence another even before there is any contact between the two, suggests that there exists what may be termed a 'region of magnetic influence' round each of them. This region is usually termed a *magnetic field*. As we shall see later (p. 146) magnetic fields also exist in the neighbourhood of wires carrying an electric current, a fact which has many important applications.

MAKING MAGNETS

If a specimen of magnetic, but unmagnetized, substance (such as steel) is stroked repeatedly in one direction with one end of a bar magnet, it will, itself, become magnetized. However, this is not a very reliable technique. Nowadays a specimen will be magnetized by placing it inside a long coil of wire (a *solenoid*), through which an electric current can be passed. Within limits (see p. 79), the higher the current, the stronger the magnetization remaining in the specimen when the current is switched off. The *direction* of the magnetization (i.e. the polarity of the magnet produced) will be determined by the *direction* of the current in the coil.

SOME IMPORTANT MAGNETIC EXPERIMENTS

The experiments which are about to be described illustrate some very important magnetic phenomena, the results of which will be discussed in some detail after dealing with the experiments themselves.

Differences in the Magnetic Behaviour of Soft Iron and Steel

A bar of soft iron is placed within a solenoid and the current is switched on. A heap of iron filings is placed near one of the projecting ends of the bar. It is found that a large bunch of filings is attracted to the magnetic pole formed at that end, indicating that the soft iron has become strongly magnetized. If now the current is switched off, almost the whole of the iron filings which were clinging to the bar fall away again, showing that the majority of the soft iron's magnetism is present only so long as the current flows; a small amount of it only remains after switching off the current.

The experiment is now repeated using a steel bar in place of the soft iron one, the same current being passed through the solenoid. Iron filings are again attracted in a bunch at the end of the bar, but the number attracted is in this case found to be smaller, showing that although the steel bar has become magnetized, the degree of magnetization induced in it for the same magnetizing current is less than in the case of soft iron. On the other hand, when the current is switched off again the majority of the iron filings are found to remain clinging to the steel. Thus although steel is not so readily magnetized as soft iron, it nevertheless retains more of its magnetism when the magnetizing influence is removed. It is usual to sum up these facts by stating that the *magnetic susceptibility* of soft iron is greater than that of steel, whereas the *retentivity* of steel is greater than that of iron.

These differing properties must be taken into account in the choice of material for different types of magnetic device. Thus for a *permanent magnet*, one which is required to retain strong magnetization over a long period even, for instance, under mechanical vibration (see p. 80), a material with a very high retentivity is chosen. Hard steels, particularly alloys containing cobalt and nickel, are most suitable for this purpose.

On the other hand there are many applications where *electro-magnets* are used. Here a coil is wound on a magnetic core so that when an electric current is passed through the coil, the core is magnetized, but if the core is of soft iron it will lose its magnetism as soon as the current in the coil is switched off. This facility of 'switching on and off' the magnetism in a soft iron core is the basis of all the relays and contactors which are so widely used in X-ray units and other electrical equipment (e.g. telephone exchanges) for switching circuits from a distance or in dangerous places, or for the switching of high voltages (see p. 153).

The Existence of Magnetic 'Saturation'

If a bar of soft iron is placed in a solenoid and the current in the coil is increased *gradually* from zero to very high values, it is found that the amount of iron filings attracted to the end of the bar does not go on increasing indefinitely. This and more refined experiments indicate that there is a limit to the amount of magnetism which may be induced in a given piece of magnetic material, that there exists, in fact, a 'saturation' point.

Splitting of a Bar Magnet into Two or More Pieces

We have already seen that if a bar magnet is dipped into iron filings, the latter cling mainly to its two ends where the magnetism in the bar appears to be concentrated (Fig. 29a). Very few filings are attracted to the region between the two poles. If such a bar is divided into two parts, however, and the separate parts are tested again by means of iron

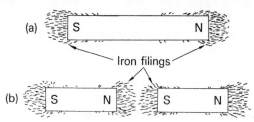

Fig. 29. When a bar magnet is broken, two separate magnets are formed.

filings, it is found that strong magnetic poles have appeared at the two ends on either side of the break (Fig. 29b). By suspending the two parts so that they can swing freely in a horizontal plane it can easily be shown that each possesses a north and south pole—in fact that each has become a complete magnet. The same would be found to be true whatever the number of parts into which the original magnet was divided —each part would be found to behave separately as a complete magnet.

Methods of Effecting Demagnetization

At red heat an ordinary magnet is found to lose its magnetic properties; these return on cooling, but the specimen is then in the unmagnetized state. Repeated hammering is also found to destroy magnetism. Neither of these methods can of course be used if the magnetized specimen (e.g. a watch) is to remain undamaged. The method of demagnetization adopted then is to place the object in a solenoid and reverse the direction of the coil current many times, whilst reducing the strength of this current to zero. The object is then magnetized in one polarity and then in the reverse polarity, each time to a slightly less extent corresponding to the lower current, until finally it is left with no residual magnetism.

THE THEORY OF FERRO-MAGNETISM

As stated at the beginning of the chapter, magnetism is not an isolated phenomenon, and we shall see later (p. 146) that with any electric current there is always an associated magnetic field. The structure of the atom is discussed in greater detail on p. 90, but it may be pointed out here that within every atom there are tiny negatively charged particles (or *electrons*) in rapid motion, and it would be expected therefore that magnetic fields will be associated with these 'atomic' currents. In general there is no *nett* magnetic effect, but for a few so-called *ferro-magnetic* materials, which are crystalline in structure, there is an interaction between the atoms so that (as a result of the *spins* of the electrons rather than their orbital motions) these atoms possess a natural magnetic effect. The atoms are in groups having the same direction of magnetization and forming what Weiss called 'domains', but the directions of magnetization of the different domains within the material are arranged at random, so that the specimen as a whole does not, in general, show any natural magnetization.

However, when the specimen is subjected to an external magnetic field during the process of magnetization, the directions of magnetization of more and more of the domains are gradually brought into line with the magnetizing field.* The random arrangement of the direction of magnetization of the domains no longer holds, and the specimen shows

* It must be stressed that there is no alignment of the atoms themselves, but only of the effective direction of magnetization of the domains.

a nett magnetization which reaches a maximum when all the domains are aligned with the external field, thus accounting for the phenomenon of magnetic saturation (p. 79). The ease with which this alignment can be carried out and the magnitude of the resultant saturation magnetization (the susceptibility, p. 78) might be expected to depend on the type of atom, the presence of any traces of impurity, and also on the crystal structure. Thus the theory can provide an explanation for the variations in magnetic properties of different forms and alloys of iron and steel.

It is only at the ends of the magnet that the external magnetic effects are observed (i.e. at the poles—p. 77). This can be more easily appreciated if each domain is considered as equivalent to a tiny bar magnet—which is not, of course, really the case. Then, as shown in Fig. 30a, each

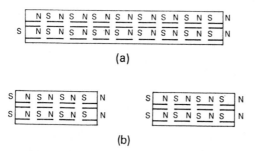

(a)

(b)

Fig. 30a. In a magnet, each domain north pole has near it the south pole of another domain, and it is only at the ends that 'free' poles are found.

Fig. 30b. When broken, the two faces at the break will show end effects (i.e. free poles) as did the original specimen.

domain north pole has near it the south pole of another domain, and it is only at the ends of the specimen that 'free' poles are to be found— north poles at one end and south poles at the other. From this same Fig. 30a it can be seen why, when a magnet is broken into two, both pieces are found to be complete magnets (p. 79). Such a break obviously goes between (and does not split) the atoms, the domains themselves not being in any way rigid structures but only groups of atoms with similar directions of magnetization. Thus the two faces of the break will show 'end' effects (due to the free poles of the end domains) as did the original specimen, and the two pieces will each have a north and a south pole as shown in Fig. 30b.

The normal (unmagnetized) arrangement of the domains within a specimen corresponds to a state of minimum energy of the material, and work must be done to align the directions of magnetization. Thus the material will always tend to resume the original state and become demagnetized. It is to variations in the ease and rapidity with which this return can take place that we may attribute differences in retentivity between various types of magnetic material (p. 78). If the specimen is hammered, the mechanical impulses provide energy which hastens the process of demagnetization.

If the specimen is heated above a certain temperature known as the *Curie temperature* of the material, the increased thermal movement of the atoms destroys the normal interaction between them which provides their natural magnetization, and so destroys the magnetic properties of the material. On cooling, the ferro-magnetic properties of the material are restored, but it will be in the unmagnetized state (p. 80).

LINES OF FORCE IN A MAGNETIC FIELD

The following experiments can be performed to illustrate the meaning of the term *magnetic line of force*.

A steel knitting needle is magnetized, and one end of it—that at which the north pole is situated—is pushed through a cork in such way that the needle will float vertically in water with this end just above the surface. It is floated in water contained in a tank or large trough filled nearly to the brim, and a strong bar magnet is placed along the edge of the tank. The arrangement is illustrated in Fig. 31a. Now it is obvious that it is impossible to obtain an *isolated* north pole by cutting off the end of a bar magnet at which its north pole is situated, for we know that the result is not an isolated north pole but two complete magnets. However, for practical purposes, with the arrangement described, the presence of the south pole of the knitting needle may be neglected, since it is at a comparatively large distance below the surface of the water. The floating needle therefore behaves roughly as though it *were* an isolated north pole.

The upper end of it is placed near the north pole of the bar magnet. Since these are like poles, repulsion occurs, and the needle moves away. The further it gets from the north pole of the bar magnet, the less the force of repulsion becomes, and the more (relatively) is the force of attraction exerted on it by the south pole of the bar magnet. The path taken by the floating magnet thus gradually curves round towards the south pole of the bar magnet, at which it eventually terminates. A slightly different starting point results in a somewhat different path but of the same general shape. A number of the paths traced out by the floating needle are shown in Fig. 31b.

The magnetic field surrounding a bar magnet may be thought of as being mapped out by such a pattern of lines. Each line may be termed a *magnetic line of force*, being defined as any path which will be traced out by an isolated north pole free to move in the magnetic field. It is obvious that the direction of (i.e. the *tangent to*) the line of force at any point gives the direction of the force which would act on any isolated north

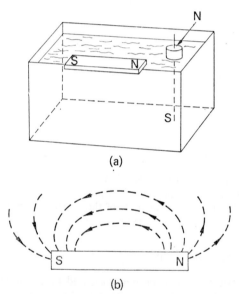

Fig. 31. Experiment to demonstrate the concept of magnetic lines of force.

pole placed at that point. The definition implies that any given line of force must begin on a north pole and ultimately terminate on a south pole. It also implies that no two lines of force may cross, for if they did it would mean that an isolated north pole at the point common to the two lines would have a choice of direction, which is contrary to experience. This problem may be dealt with in another manner. Suppose two bar magnets are placed near to each other so that lines of force due to one overlap lines of force due to the other at some points. Then at such a point as *P* (Fig. 32) we have apparently two lines of force which cross. Now each line of force represents the direction of a force which would act on an isolated north pole placed at *P*. Thus, a north pole placed at *P* will be acted on by two forces in directions *PQ* and *PR* respectively. We know, however, that two such forces may be combined into a single *resultant* force *PS* by means of the Parallelogram of Forces (p. 10). It follows that two or more magnetic fields, when superimposed, combine to form what may be termed a *resultant* magnetic field; and it is in this resultant field that no lines of force will cross.

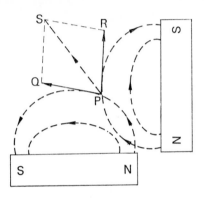

Fig. 32. A north pole placed at *P* will be acted upon by two forces in the direction of *PQ* and *PR* respectively, which combine to give a single resultant force *PS* representing the direction and magnitude of the resultant magnetic field at the point.

Some Typical Magnetic Fields

All these magnetic fields can be demonstrated in a simple fashion by placing a thin card over the arrangement of magnets concerned and covering the card lightly and evenly with fine iron filings. If the card is then tapped gently the filings set themselves along the lines of force to form a pattern of the magnetic field. Thus, for a simple bar magnet the pattern shown in Fig. 33a is obtained.

For two bar magnets it is to be seen from Fig. 33b that where there is attraction, the lines of force pass across the intervening space from the one pole to the other (unlike) pole, whereas in the case where there is repulsion (Fig. 33c), the lines of force move away from each other in the region between the two (like) poles. At some point (*P* in Fig. 33c) between the two poles the magnetic fields due to the two magnets are equal and opposite and therefore cancel out. This point is therefore referred to as a *null point*.

In Fig. 33d the effect of placing a piece of soft iron in a magnetic field is seen. The lines of force are concentrated into the soft iron, preferring to go through it rather than through the surrounding air. This effect is attributed to the fact that the so-called *magnetic permeability* of iron is high.

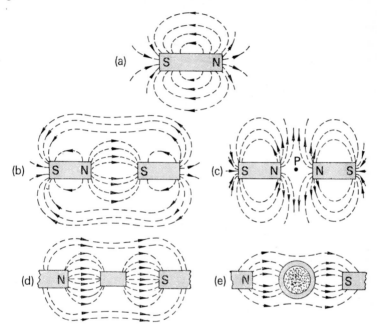

Fig. 33. Some typical magnetic fields:
(a) a simple bar magnet,
(b) two bar magnets with unlike poles adjacent,
(c) two bar magnets with like poles adjacent,
(d) the effect of placing a piece of soft iron in a magnetic field,
(e) the effect of placing a soft iron ring in a magnetic field.

In Fig. 33e the iron is in the form of a flat ring, and in this case it is found that the iron filings on the area of card over the space inside the ring show little or no tendency to align themselves in any particular direction, indicating that the space within the ring is more or less screened by it from the surrounding magnetic field. It follows that to screen, for instance, an electrical instrument from external magnetic fields, it should be placed inside a box of soft iron, or other material of very high permeability, such as the special alloy known as 'mu-metal'. Such screening may in some cases be necessary for meters or relays, whilst, for instance, television tubes may need a close fitting cover of mu-metal to prevent magnetic pick-up from the other electrical apparatus in the set.

This concentration of the magnetic field into a material of high permeability is also used to assist the retention of magnetization in permanent magnets. If left on their own such magnets do gradually tend to lose their magnetization. A better plan is to store them in pairs, as shown in Fig. 34, with unlike poles adjacent and joined by pieces of soft iron which are referred to as *keepers*. The lines of force running from the one magnet to the other are then concentrated in the keepers and tend to maintain the orientation of the domains within the magnets.

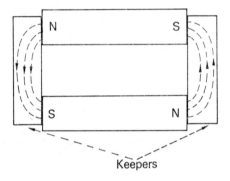

Fig. 34. Storage of bar magnets with the aid of soft iron keepers.

HYSTERESIS

It has already been explained that if a specimen of iron or steel is placed inside a solenoid and the current in the solenoid is gradually increased, the magnetization of the specimen will also increase until the magnet becomes 'saturated'. Plotting the magnetization of the specimen against the current (which is a measure of the magnetizing field) therefore gives a curve such as *ABC* in Fig. 35a, *C* corresponding to the maximum (*saturation*) value of the magnetization. Now if the current is reduced the magnetization falls, but even with zero current some magnetization remains in the specimen. This change is shown by the curve *CDE*, and *AE* is a measure of the retentivity (p. 78). The magnetization can be reduced to zero by increasing the coil current with the reverse connection to the battery (curve *EF*), this current, represented by *AF*,

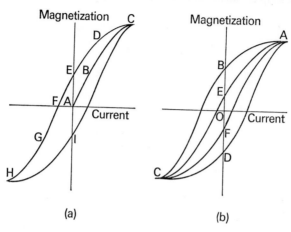

Fig. 35.
(a) Hysteresis curve for a specimen of iron.
(b) Hysteresis curves: *ABCDA* steel, and *AECFA* soft iron.

being a measure of the so-called *coercive force* necessary for demagnetization. After this a further increase in the current in the reverse direction magnetizes the specimen again up to saturation, but with the reverse polarity (*FGH*). Reduction to zero, reversal and increase of the current again in the original direction completes the magnetization curve along *HI* to *C*, and further current reversals would give magnetization changes corresponding to the loop *CDEFGHIC*. It will be noticed that during this cycle the change in magnetization always lags behind the change in solenoid current. This phenomenon is known as *hysteresis*, and the curve as a *hysteresis curve*. Although all magnetic samples show the same general form of curve the shape of the loop depends on the type of material. Thus in Fig. 35b *ABCDA* would correspond to a sample of steel (with a high retentivity *OB* and *OD*), and *AECFA* to a specimen of soft iron (where very little magnetization *OE* and *OF* is left when the current is switched off). Without going into great detail it can be said that the *area* within the hysteresis loop is a measure of the work done in orientating and reorientating the direction of magnetization of the domains during the cycle of magnetization. In instruments where magnetic material is subject to such cyclic changes (e.g. in the core of a transformer), this work represents an energy loss. Thus, to minimize this loss a magnetic material is chosen which has a hysteresis loop enclosing only a small area (e.g. soft iron or silicon steel).

CHAPTER 6

Electrostatics

INTRODUCTION

It has been known from very early times that *amber* can, after being rubbed, attract certain light objects to itself. It is said to be *electrified* (or *charged* with *electricity*), and the phenomenon is termed *electrification by friction*.

In the sixteenth century Gilbert classified substances according to whether they behaved like amber or not, calling those which did *electrics* and those which did not *non-electrics*. Gilbert's 'electrics' we now call *insulators*, and his so-called 'non-electrics', *conductors*. In the case of conductors, an electric charge placed on one part of it can flow easily to any other part. In insulators, on the other hand, this process is very much more difficult.

The Two States of Electrification

If an *ebonite* rod which has been rubbed with fur to electrify it is suspended in a stirrup from a fine thread (Fig. 36a), and a second ebonite rod, electrified in the same manner, is brought near to it, a force of repulsion is found to exist between the two, as is evidenced by the fact that the first rod moves away from the second as the latter approaches.

It can be demonstrated in a similar manner that two *glass* rods, electrified by rubbing them with silk, also repel each other (Fig. 36b).

On the other hand, if a glass rod rubbed with silk is brought near to a suspended ebonite rod which has been rubbed with fur (Fig. 36c), *attraction* is found to take place.

These results may be described in a simple manner by *postulating* that there are two states of electrification, one of which may (arbitrarily) be termed *positive* and the other (in an equally arbitrary manner) *negative*. The words *positive* and *negative* are merely labels, and their use here is not to be confused with the mathematical associations of these terms.

Thus we say that the ebonite rubbed with fur is *negatively* charged, and
the glass rubbed with silk *positively* charged, and it is then seen that the

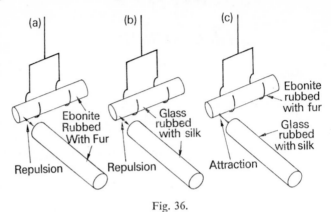

Fig. 36.

experimental results just described can be summed up in the simple
statement '*like charges repel, unlike charges attract*' (sometimes referred to as the First Law of Electrostatics, cf. the First Law of Magnetism, p. 77).

INTRODUCTION TO ATOMIC STRUCTURE:
THE ELECTRON THEORY OF ELECTRIFICATION

The theory that all substances are composed of tiny particles called
'atoms' has already been mentioned (p. 1). In the early form of this
theory it was considered that atoms themselves were indivisible, and
that for this reason they represented the smallest unit into which matter
could be divided. However, it is now known that, far from being indivisible, atoms have a structure of their own, comparatively simple
in the case of some elements, and extremely complex in the case of
others. Ninety-two different kinds of atoms (i.e. ninety-two different
elements) occur in nature, of which the gas *hydrogen* has the simplest
atomic structure, and the metal *uranium* the most intricate. Of recent
years, a number of 'man-made' elements, heavier than uranium, have
been added to the naturally-occurring ones, and are referred to as the
trans-uranic elements.

   The kind of terms in which we depict the structure of atoms depends
to some extent on the phenomena which we seek to explain in this way.

As each new experimental observation is made, so, to a greater or lesser degree, the mental picture which we have of the atom itself must change. Here, with our immediate study of electrification in mind, we must content ourselves with a description, in deliberately simplified terms of a few of the least complex atoms, and it must always be remembered that the picture thus drawn, whilst adequate for our purpose, would be quite inadequate as an explanation of many phenomena which do not concern us here.*

In general terms, then, we may consider any atom to be like a miniature solar system, the total distance across which is of the order of one hundred millionth of a centimetre (10^{-8} cm). At the centre is a *nucleus* (analogous to the sun) which is *positively* charged. The diameter of this nucleus is of the order of only 10^{-12} cm and with it is associated almost all the *mass* of the atom. Round this, in particular orbits, revolve very light particles known as *electrons* (analogous to the planets), which are *negatively* charged. The simplest atom of all is that of hydrogen, whose nucleus has a single electron revolving round it.

Now it has been found that simple relationships exist among the magnitudes of the *charges* carried by the nuclei of different elements, these being in all cases simple multiples of that carried by the hydrogen nucleus (or *proton*, as the hydrogen nucleus is called). Thus, if we call the charge carried by the hydrogen nucleus $+1$ unit, the charge carried by the nucleus of the next simplest atom, helium, is $+2$ units, that carried by the lithium nucleus $+3$ units, and so on up to the uranium nucleus, which carries a charge of $+92$ units. This number of positive charges carried by the nucleus is known as the *atomic number* of that particular element.

Now in its normal state an atom is electrically *neutral*, and hence the total amounts of positive and negative charge which it carries must be exactly equal. The positive charge is carried by the *nucleus*, and the negative charge by the *electrons* revolving round it; and since, in fact, each electron carries 1 unit of negative charge, it follows that, in order to balance out the positive charge on the nucleus, *the number of electrons revolving round the latter in the normal state of the atom must be equal to the number of units of positive charge carried by the nucleus* (i.e. the *atomic number*). For example, the hydrogen atom, the nucleus of which carries

---

* The concept of atomic structure, some account of which follows, is based on the model first propounded by Bohr. A more comprehensive account of atomic theory would involve, among other things, 'wave mechanics', which is outside our present scope.

1 unit of positive charge, normally has 1 electron revolving round it. The helium atom on the other hand has 2 units of positive charge on its nucleus, and will therefore normally have 2 electrons revolving round it, the lithium nucleus 3 electrons, and so on.

If an atom acquires one or more electrons in excess of its normal complement, it will have a surplus of negative charge, and will, in fact, be *negatively charged*. Conversely, an atom *losing* one or more of its normal complement of electrons, will be *deficient* in negative charge, and will have a surplus of *positive* charge: it will be *positively* charged.

This process of losing electrons, or of gaining extra ones, goes on between the atoms of two substances rubbed together, and explains why they become 'electrified'. For example, when ebonite is rubbed with fur, the fur *loses* electrons to the ebonite. Thus the ebonite, initially electrically neutral, has a *surplus* of electrons, and is now negatively charged; whilst the fur, having a *deficit* of electrons, must have become *positively* charged.

In a similar way we may say that when glass is rubbed with silk, the *glass* loses electrons (to the silk), the former becoming *positively* charged, and the latter negatively charged.

In general, in any process of electrification brought about by placing together two dissimilar surfaces in intimate contact, there is a transfer of electrons from one surface to the other. The direction in which the transfer takes place depends on the particular substances involved, and is not governed by any simple rule. Everyday examples are the electrification of the hair (when in a dry state) by a plastic comb, and the charges produced by friction on silk, nylon, woollen and other garments.

Insulators and Conductors

In *conductors* the electrons in orbits furthest from the nucleus can move easily from one atom to another, i.e. they can flow easily from one part of the conductor to another (they are, in fact, virtually 'free' electrons —see also p. 127), whereas in *insulators*, although it is possible for electrons to be removed from, or added to, an atom by such a process as friction, normally even those in the outermost orbits of the atom are much more difficult to dislodge, i.e. they cannot pass easily from one atom to another.

ELECTRIC CURRENTS

A flow of electric charges is generally referred to as an '*electric current*'. Under appropriate conditions electric currents can be made to flow in solids, liquids and gases. No translational movement of whole atoms can take place in the case of solids, so that (since the positive electricity resides entirely on the nuclei of atoms) only the carriers of negative electricity, i.e. the electrons, can move from one part to another of a solid. In liquids and gases, in which whole atoms (and therefore atomic nuclei) are mobile, both positive and negative electricity can flow.

The Direction of an Electric Current

It became conventional to refer to a flow of positive electricity from one point *A*, say, to another point *B* as an *electric current* from *A* to *B*. A little thought will indicate that from the electrical point of view, a flow of *negative* charges from *B* to *A* is exactly equivalent to this. Since in solids only electrons can flow, it follows that when, on the above convention, we refer to a flow of current in a certain direction *what is actually occurring is a flow of electrons in the opposite direction*. This is true, for example, of all the metal wiring of which electrical circuits are largely composed, and this fact must always be borne in mind when referring to the conventional direction of current flow.

The earth, as a large conductor, may be thought of as an enormous reservoir of electrons making up any deficiency of, or taking any surplus away from, an object connected to it by a conducting path. This is what was meant by saying that a charge 'leaked away' to earth; for whether a body has a deficiency of electrons made up, or a surplus of them taken away, it becomes electrically neutral once again, or *discharged*, when it is connected to earth.

Further reference will be made to this matter in the discussion on electric potential (p. 97).

ELECTRIC FIELDS: ELECTRIC LINES OF FORCE

Just as there is a magnetic 'field' in the neighbourhood of a magnetic pole (see p. 77), so also is there an *electric* field in the neighbourhood of an electric charge, and, corresponding to the so-called *magnetic line of force* by means of which magnetic fields may be depicted, we have *electric* lines of force.

An electric line of force may be defined as any path which would be taken by a positive charge, free to move under the influence of the field (cf. the definition of magnetic lines of force, p. 82). Typical electric fields (in a single plane) are shown in Fig. 37. The following observations may be made with regard to these fields:

(a) The lines of force all *begin* on a positive charge.

(b) In point of fact, they all end on a negative charge, although this

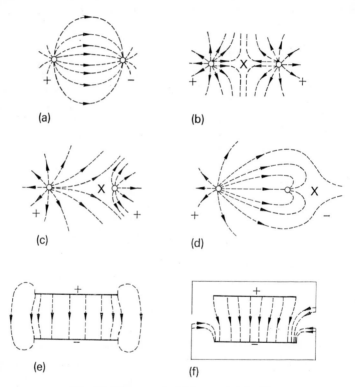

Fig. 37. Electrostatic fields associated with

(a) two equal, unlike charges,
(b) two equal, like charges,
(c) two unequal, like charges,
(d) two unequal and unlike charges,
(f) two parallel plates carrying equal and unlike charges,
(e) a 'free-air' ionization chamber.

may not be seen to be the case for all the lines shown. This is because, in cases where *both* charges considered are positive, the *negative* charges on which the lines of force terminate will be on surrounding objects such as the walls of the room (such charges being said to be 'induced' on these objects, see p. 101).

(c) All the lines of force meet the charged surfaces at right angles, which is in fact always true when the charges involved are *at rest, and situated on a conductor*. This is a matter of some importance, and will be referred to again.

(d) Between two like charges there is a point X (Fig. 37b and c) at which the resultant force on a third charge would be zero. Such a point is called a *null* point (cf. p. 85), and for obvious reasons no lines of force pass through it. The null point is midway between equal like charges (Fig. 37b), but nearer to the weaker charge in the case of unequal charges (Fig. 37c). A little thought will show that there must also be a null point *beyond* the weaker of two *un*like and *un*-equal charges at which the force due to the nearer (weaker) charge is counterbalanced by the oppositely directed force due to the larger (and more distant) charge (Fig. 37d).

(e) Fig. 37e shows the lines of force in a plane at right angles to two identical parallel plates carrying equal but unlike charges. Fig. 37f shows the sort of thing which can happen to the field when the two plates are situated in an earthed metal box having (circular) holes in either end. Such an arrangement corresponds to a type of standard ionization chamber (known as a parallel-plate or 'free-air' chamber) used for X-ray exposure standardization, and study of the associated electrostatic field distribution is therefore of great importance.

Resultant Electrostatic Field

We have seen (p. 84) that no two *magnetic* lines of force can cross, since at such a point of intersection in superimposed fields the two lines, representing as they do the directions of two *forces*, may be combined (by the Parallelogram of Forces) into a single line of force: and this can be done at all such points. This argument will obviously hold good for electrostatic fields also (Fig. 38).

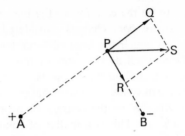

Fig. 38. Resultant electrostatic field. A positive charge at *P* is repelled in the direction *PQ* and attracted in the direction *PR*, so that the resultant force is in the direction *PS*.

THE ELECTROSTATIC UNIT OF CHARGE

This is defined as the magnitude of that charge which exerts a force of 1 dyne on an equal charge placed 1 cm from it *in vacuo*.

The force between electric charges can be profoundly influenced by the medium between them (which, if it fills the space between the charges, must of necessity be an insulating material). Such a material is, in these circumstances, generally referred to as a *dielectric*. The effect on the force acting when air at atmospheric pressure is the dielectric is small enough to be quite negligible for almost all practical purposes. Thus, although the definition of unit charge specifies a *vacuum* between the two charges concerned, the force will be practically unmodified by the presence of air. Where the effects of the dielectric on the force acting are not negligible, they are taken into account by means of a factor (usually represented by *k*), known as the *dielectric constant* of the medium (see below).

The Law of Force Between Electric Charges

This force is proportional to the product of the magnitudes of the charges, and *inversely* proportional to the *square* of the distance between them, being given by the equation

$$\text{force (in dynes)} = \frac{q_1 q_2}{kd^2},$$

where q_1 and q_2 are the magnitudes of the two charges (in electrastatic units), *d* is the distance (in cm) between them, and *k* is the dielectric *constant* of the intervening medium. Values of the dielectric constant for some common insulating materials are given in Table IV.

TABLE IV

Material	Dielectric Constant
Ebonite	2·8
Mica	6
Paper	2
Paraffin Wax	2
Rubber	2·2
Transformer Oil	4·5
Air	1

So far as the variation of the force with distance is concerned, this is spoken of as an *inverse square* relationship, which also occurs in a number of other contexts in physics (see, for instance p. 225).

Electric Field Strength or Intensity

At any point in an electrostatic field, the field strength may be measured in terms of the force which the field produces on a unit positive charge placed at the point considered. Thus the field is said to be 1 electrostatic unit if it exerts a force of 1 dyne on unit charge placed at the given point.

ELECTRICAL POTENTIAL AND POTENTIAL DIFFERENCE

A conductor *A* is to be considered at a higher potential than conductor *B* if, when the two are connected together, a (conventional) *current flows from A to B* to achieve the equalization of potentials.* On this basis it is easy to see that zero on the potential scale is to be identified with *earth* potential. For, when an isolated positively charged conductor (i.e. one *deficient* in electrons) is connected to earth, its deficiency of electrons is made up by a flow of electrons (i.e. negative charges) from earth to the conductor: that is, the conventional *current* flow is from the conductor to earth. Therefore an isolated positively charged conductor must be considered as being *above* earth potential. Similarly, when an isolated negatively charged conductor (i.e. one having a surplus of

* Cf. the flow of gas between two containers connected together to equalize the two gas pressures.

electrons) is connected to earth, its surplus of electrons flows away *to* earth, constituting a conventional current flow from earth to the conductor. Thus the potential of an isolated negatively charged conductor must be considered to be *below* earth potential. It follows that earth potential corresponds to zero on our scale, being a kind of *standard level* of potential to which all other electric potentials can be referred, in much the same way as heights (and depths) are referred to sea level.

We could summarize these observations on electric potential by stating that *the potential of a conductor is the electrical condition associated with it which determines in which direction an electric current flows when the conductor is connected to earth* (from body to earth for a body having a positive potential, and from earth to the body for a body having a negative potential).

Free and Induced Potential

The potential imparted to an isolated conductor *by its own charge* may be called its *free* potential. Now an insulated *un*charged conductor can also acquire a potential (positive or negative) by virtue of its *proximity* to a charged body or bodies (easily shown by the fact that when such an uncharged conductor is connected to earth a current flow to, or from, earth can be demonstrated). Such a potential, acquired by an uncharged body by virtue of its proximity to a charged one, may be referred to as an *induced* potential. The nearer the uncharged body is placed to the charged body, the closer does its induced potential approximate to the free potential of the charged body.*

Conductors as Equipotential Surfaces

It has been seen above that when two conductors initially at different potentials are connected together, a current flows along the conducting link until the potentials of the two conductors are equalized. Now different parts of the *same* conductor may be considered from a similar standpoint, and it follows at once that the whole of the surface of a conductor *on which the charges have settled down* (i.e. are at rest) must be at the same potential—it is, in fact, an *equipotential surface*. If, by some means, a difference in potential *is* momentarily produced between

---

* There being, however, some lowering of this free potential, brought about by the approach of the uncharged conductor (see p. 111).

different parts of the surface of the same conductor, then currents must flow over the surface until the redistribution of charges brought about in this way *exactly counterbalances the effects of the agent tending to establish and maintain such a potential difference.* It follows that although the *potential* on the surface of such a conductor is everywhere the same, the *charge* on its surface may not be by any means evenly distributed. In fact (apart from conductors considered theoretically to be of infinite extent) the *isolated* charged sphere is the only case where an even distribution of charge accompanies the equipotential condition, a result which follows directly from the symmetry of the arrangement.

INDUCTIVE DISPLACEMENT

Consider a positively charged object (indicated by a sphere P in Fig. 39a), and suppose two small, insulated uncharged conductors (indicated by spheres A and B) are placed nearby, as shown. For convenience, the diagram also incorporates a rough graphical indication of the variation of potential with distance measured in the direction PAB. To begin with, this will be somewhat as shown in Fig. 39a. P has some definite positive potential V, due to its charge, and the potential in the direction of A and B falls off steadily with distance, as shown. The horizontal parts of the curve above each of the spheres indicates the equipotential condition of their surfaces. A and B will each acquire an induced positive potential owing to their proximity to P, but since A is nearer to P than B is, its potential will be higher ($V_1 > V_2$). It follows that if A and B are connected together by a conducting link, a 'current' will flow from A to B* until A and B are at the same, uniform, positive potential V_3 (intermediate between V_1 and V_2). Thus B is left with a deficit of negative charge, i.e. it is *positively* charged, whilst A has a surplus of negative charge. Taken together, A and B are still electrically neutral; no charge has been given to them or taken from them, but there has been a *displacement* of charges to establish the equipotential condition. The plot of potential against distance will now be somewhat as shown in Fig. 39b.

This redistribution of charges is called *inductive displacement*, and its existence may be demonstrated by subsequently breaking the connection

---

* In practice, of course, *electrons* (negative charges) flow from B to A (see p. 93).

between *A* and *B* (thus isolating the displaced charges) and bringing each in turn up to (a) a positively charged pith ball suspended by an insulating thread, and (b) a similarly arranged *negatively* charged pith ball. *A* is found to repel the negatively charged ball, and *B* the positively charged ball, showing them to be negatively and positively charged respectively.

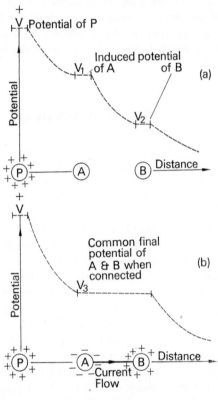

Fig. 39.

(a) Variation of potential near a positively charged sphere *P*. *A* and *B* are insulated uncharged conducting spheres.

(b) Variation of potential near a positively charged sphere *P*, with spheres *A* and *B* connected together.

The attraction of uncharged objects by a charged object is explained by inductive displacement. Thus, whether the object is positively or negatively charged, it produces a force of attraction on the *unlike* charge which separates out on the *near* side of the uncharged object, and a force of repulsion on the *like* charge which separates out on the *far* side. Since the force of attraction is associated with the *near* side, it will obviously predominate.

From the above analysis it is also seen that the presence of an uncharged conductor will always *lower* the magnitude of the potential (positive or negative) of a neighbouring *charged* conductor, once again owing to the predominating effect of the opposite sign of charge which separates out on the near side of the uncharged conductor. This phenomenon is of basic importance in analysing the action of an electric capacitor (see p. 112).

Electrification by Induction

We have already seen (p. 89) how insulators and insulated conductors can be electrified by friction. We shall now describe a more elegant method, known as electrification by induction, which is in many ways more useful, and is of considerable practical importance.

Suppose we wish to charge an insulated metal sphere by means of a positively charged rod. First, then, the positively charged rod is brought near to the insulated sphere (Fig. 40a), thereby imparting to the sphere a certain positive potential, as indicated. The sphere is then earthed (e.g. by touching it with the finger). Since the sphere had a positive potential, a 'current' must flow from it to earth (meaning that, in fact, *electrons* flow from earth to the sphere), *until the negative charge which the sphere acquires in this way produces a free negative potential which exactly counterbalances the induced potential due to the presence of the charged rod.* The sphere is then at earth potential, and the current ceases (Fig. 40b). If now the earth connection is broken, and *subsequently* the positively charged rod is removed, the sphere is left with a surplus of electrons, i.e. it is *negatively* charged (Fig. 40c).

Summarizing, it is to be noted that:

(a) the charge acquired is *opposite* in sign to that of the charge used to induce it,

(b) there are four essential steps in the induction process. These steps are as follows.

(i) The charged object is brought near to the body to be charged.

(ii) The latter is earthed.

(iii) The earth connection is broken.

(iv) The original charged object is removed.

Give a brief account (with diagrams) of the above four steps, when the charge initially available is a *negative* one.

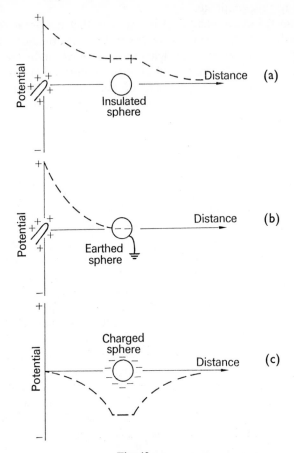

Fig. 40.

(a) A positively charged rod imparts a positive potential to an insulated conducting sphere nearby.

(b) Current flows to earth to reduce the potential of the sphere to zero.

(c) With the earth connection broken and the charged rod removed, the sphere is left negatively charged.

Some mention is worthwhile here of a simple radiological application of charge induction.* Its purpose is to induce a standardizing charge

* See L. A. W. Kemp, *Brit. Journ. Radiol.*, 1951, *24*, 211.

on the collecting electrode of an ionization chamber, used for X-ray and gamma-ray dosimetry. Such a chamber is typically of 'thimble' form (Fig. 41), consisting of a central insulated collecting electrode (a

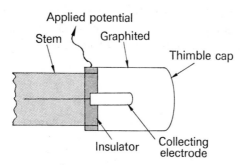

Fig. 41. A 'thimble' ionization chamber.

thin wire or rod) surrounded by a thimble-shaped cap of conducting material whose inner surface is coated with a conducting material (e.g. graphite). In normal use, for the measurement of X-rays or gamma-rays, a potential difference is applied between the cap and the collecting electrode, causing charges released in the enclosed air volume (by the action of the radiation) to be attracted to the collecting electrode, the quantity of charge collected being a measure of the radiation to which the chamber has been exposed.

To induce a calibrating charge the cap can be made to play the role of the charged body, and the collecting electrode the object to be charged. A known potential is applied to the cap (e.g. from a battery), and the collecting electrode is then earthed by means of a key built into the instrument in conjunction with which the chamber is used. This earthing key is then opened again, at which stage the collecting electrode has a charge isolated on it, the *free* potential due to which exactly counter-balances the *induced* potential due to the charged cap. This induced potential is then eliminated by earthing the *cap* (equivalent to removing the cap to a distance), thus leaving the charge on the collecting electrode to impart an appropriate *free* potential to the electrode, which is then used for calibration purposes.

THE GOLD LEAF
ELECTROSCOPE

This is a sensitive instrument for the detection (and in certain circumstances, the measurement) of electric potentials and charges. Its invention about 1780 was responsible for forwarding considerably the study of electrostatics.

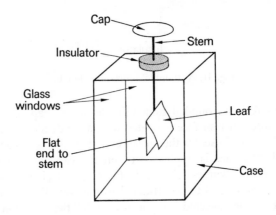

Fig. 42. A gold leaf electroscope.

A typical gold leaf electroscope is shown diagrammatically in Fig. 42. A conducting rod carrying at the top a metal 'cap', is mounted in an insulating support (the latter formerly being of rock sulphur or amber, but nowadays often one of the plastic materials such as perspex). The lower end of the conducting rod is usually flattened out, and attached to the upper edge of the flattened portion is a very thin metal leaf of, for example, gold or aluminium, which hangs limply when the electroscope is uncharged. Surrounding the lower part of the conducting stem is the case, the sides of which are of conducting material, the front and back faces usually being of glass, through which the leaf can be observed. When the instrument is to be used for measurement purposes a low-power microscope is mounted opposite the front window so that the leaf can be observed (edgewise) through it. The actual extent of the leaf's movement can be measured by means of an 'eyepiece scale' incorporated in the microscope.

The metal part of the case plays an essential part in the functioning of the electroscope, as may be seen from the following experiments. In normal use the metal case is earthed and so its potential is zero. The cap, stem and leaf, constituting a single insulated conductor, are influenced by the proximity of a charged body, their potential being raised by a positive charge or lowered by a negative charge in the neighbourhood. In each case the metal leaf is found to move away from the stem, it 'diverges'.

Now consider the cap, stem and leaf connected to earth and the case insulated from it. As a charged body is brought up, a potential is induced on the metal case and the leaf again diverges. But if the electroscope is insulated from earth and the cap, stem and leaf *connected to the case*, whatever potential is induced, there can be no potential difference between the leaf and the case. Under these conditions the proximity of a charged body does *not* cause the leaf to diverge.

Thus, the essential condition to produce a divergence of the leaf is that a potential *difference* exists between it and the metal case. The greater the potential difference, the greater will be the force acting to raise the leaf. With the case earthed, this potential difference will be equal to the potential acquired by the leaf and so the electroscope can be used to compare potentials.

UNITS OF POTENTIAL

Work must be done to build up the potential of a charged body, for each small element of charge (after the first) must be brought up against the force of repulsion exerted on it by the (like) charge already there.

The higher the potential of the body the greater the amount of work done in bringing up a given charge to it. Now the charged body imparts a potential to points in space around it and again the higher the potential at the point, the greater the amount of work done in bringing up a given charge to that point.

All this suggests that potential can, in fact, be *measured* in terms of the work done in bringing up a standard charge *from a very long way off* (from 'infinity'), where it can start free of all influence and so at zero potential. Actually we consider 1 e.s. unit of positive charge and measure the work in ergs (p. 39).

Now it follows from what has already been said as to the existence of *positive* and *negative* potentials and the differences between them (p. 98), that the work referred to will be done *on* the standard charge when the potential concerned is itself *positive*, and *by* the standard charge when the potential is *negative* (for, in the first instance a force of repulsion will be operating, and in the second a force of attraction).

To sum up then: *the potential at a point is 1 e.s. unit if 1 erg of work is done on (or by) 1 e.s. unit of positive charge in being moved from infinity to the point considered (the potential being positive if the work is done on the standard charge and negative if it is done by it).* It follows at once that ($Q \times V$) ergs will be done in moving a charge of Q e.s. units from infinity to a point at which the potential is V e.s. units.

This unit of potential is, in fact, rather inconveniently large for many practical purposes, and consequently we have the *volt* (see also p. 129) as the practical unit, which is 1/300th of the e.s. unit of potential, and this corresponds to one joule (p. 39) of work being done in bringing up one coulomb (p. 129) of charge from infinity.

The Potential Difference Between Two Points

It is clear that this will be given by the difference in the amount of work done in bringing unit positive charge from infinity *up to each of the points in turn.* Numerically, this will obviously be equal to the work done in moving unit positive charge *from one point to the other.*

It should be realized that this amount of work will be independent of the path taken by the standard charge in moving from one point to the other. In fact, potential is a *scalar* quantity (cf. the fact that the work done against gravity by a man climbing a mountain is independent of the path he takes up the mountain—see p. 41).

THE MEASUREMENT OF POTENTIAL

Instruments for the measurement of potential electrostatically (i.e. without the need for a steady current flow through the measuring instrument) are called *electrometers*. The classic instrument of this type is the *quadrant* electrometer, but this is essentially a laboratory instrument and will not be discussed here, although the principle of the quadrant electrometer was employed in at least one of the earlier forms of X-ray exposure meter. The gold leaf electroscope can be adapted and used for this purpose under laboratory conditions, but is also not robust enough for routine use.

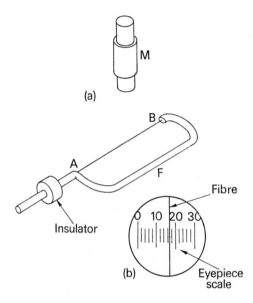

Fig. 43.
(a) Simplified diagram of a fibre electrometer.
(b) Fibre, as seen through the viewing miscroscope.

A device of interest to the student of radiology is the *fibre* electrometer, used in several well-known modern exposure meters (such as the Victoreen instrument). Essentially, it consists of a supporting frame *F* (Fig. 43a) between the ends of which is stretched a very fine conducting fibre *AB*. (In practice one end of this fibre is usually attached to a quartz fibre loop.) This system is mounted (on an insulating support) inside a metal case, so that the fibre and its supporting frame are in a horizontal plane. The fibre is viewed through a low-power microscope *M*, so that a small part of it is seen crossing the eyepiece scale of the microscope in the direction of the graduations, as shown in Fig. 43b. When a potential difference is established between the fibre and the case, the fibre bends slightly towards the case. This movement can be observed (and measured) by means of the microscope and its eyepiece scale, and a suitable calibration would enable changes in potential of objects connected to the fibre to be measured in terms of the fibre movement. In an X-ray exposure meter, however, this electrometer system is employed to measure the change in potential of the collector after the chamber has been exposed to ionising radiation, this change in potential being an indication of the amount of radiation to which the chamber has been exposed. The eyepiece scale of the instrument is therefore calibrated direct in 'roentgens', the unit of X-ray exposure.

Electrostatic voltmeters must also be included here, although these instruments are less sensitive than 'electrometers'. They are, however, direct-reading and relatively robust.

The majority of these instruments are derived from the quadrant electrometer referred to above, and their action may be explained in terms of the force of attraction which exists between unlike charges. Consider two metal plates *A* and *B* (Fig. 44a), parallel to the plane of the paper and therefore to each other, and partially overlapping, with, however, a small gap between them. Plate *A* is fixed, but the sector-shaped plate *B* can pivot about *P*, whilst remaining parallel to *A*. If now, the potential difference to be measured is applied between *A* and *B*, one plate will become positively charged and the other negatively charged, and attraction will ensue. This attraction will cause *B* to turn about the pivot *P* so that more of *B* comes opposite *A* (Fig. 44a). The movement of *B* can be controlled by a spring, so that equilibrium will be reached when the electrostatic attraction is balanced by the moment due to the spring. The greater the potential difference applied between *A* and *B*, the greater the angle through which *B* will turn before reaching the equilibrium position. Thus the angle through which *B* turns (as indicated by a pointer on a scale) can be employed as a measure of the potential difference applied between *A* and *B*. The force between the plates will be proportional to the product of the charges on them (see p. 96) which in turn will be proportional to the *square* of the applied potential difference. Thus, whilst this results in a non-linear instrument scale, it does enable the instrument to be used for the measurement of alternating potentials, since the force between the plates is one of attraction whichever way round the potential is applied.

To make the instrument more sensitive, a multiplicity of fixed and moving vanes can be employed as shown in Fig. 44, thus multiplying the deflecting force by a factor equal to the number of pairs of parallel surfaces provided in this way.

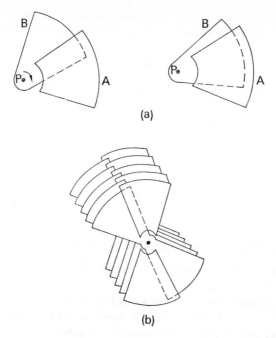

Fig. 44.
(a) Principle of the electrostatic voltmeter.
(b) Practical arrangement of vanes in an electrostatic voltmeter.

THE RELATION BETWEEN THE CHARGE ON AN ISOLATED, INSULATED CONDUCTOR, AND THE POTENTIAL WHICH IT PRODUCES: ELECTRICAL CAPACITANCE

If equal charges are placed on two isolated conductors they will produce equal potentials only if the two conductors are identical in size and shape. If one conductor has a greater size and surface area than the other, then the charge will have a greater area over which to spread itself and therefore the potential which it produces will be less (cf. the pressures produced by the same amounts of gas placed in two different-sized containers).

In fact, the *capacity* (for holding electricity) of the larger conductor is greater than that of the smaller.

By experiment it can be shown that if the charge on a given isolated conductor is doubled, its potential is doubled, and so on. That is, the potential V of the conductor is proportional to the charge Q given to it, or

$$Q = \text{constant} \times V.$$

This constant is called the *capacity* (or *capacitance*) of the conductor, and is generally indicated by C.

Thus we may write $Q = VC,$

whence $V = \dfrac{Q}{C},$

and $C = \dfrac{Q}{V}.$

Factors Affecting the Capacitance of a Conductor

The capacitance of a conductor depends on:
  (i) its size and shape,
  (ii) its position relative to other conductors,
  (iii) the medium in which it is situated, or, in the case of (ii), the medium between it and neighbouring conductors.

We shall describe in turn experiments to illustrate the effects of these factors.

(i) The cap of a gold leaf electroscope is fitted with a device which enables the surface area of the cap, stem, and leaf system to be increased at will without discharging the system. For example, a metallized balloon may be fitted which can be inflated by means of a tube of insulating material, or a metal foil 'roller blind' may be attached which can be extended by means of an insulating thread. It is found that, in these circumstances, if the electroscope is first charged, and subsequently the balloon is inflated (or the 'blind' extended) thus causing the surface over which the charge can spread to increase, the divergence of the leaf is found to *de*crease. That is, regarding the cap, stem, leaf and extensible conductor as a single, charged system, we may say that *for a given charge* the potential of the system decreases as the surface area *in*creases. But, since (see above) $Q = VC$, and since, also, Q is constant, it follows that the product VC will be constant. Hence, if the potential V is found to *decrease*, it must mean that the capacitance C has *increased*. Thus we may sum up by saying that an increase in the surface area of a conductor results in an increase in its capacitance.

So far as shape is concerned, this is to be considered in conjunction with *size*, but we may say that for a given volume the shape which provides the greatest surface area (which is not re-entrant) will also provide the greatest capacitance.

(ii) An electroscope is charged, and an uncharged metal plate, fitted with an insulating handle, is then lowered gradually towards the top cap of the electroscope. It is found that the divergence of the leaf is reduced, showing that the capacitance of the electroscope is being *increased* (see discussion under (i) above). If the insulated metal plate is earthed and the experiment repeated, the effect is found to be enhanced; that is, for a given spacing between the two plates, the increase in capacitance is made still greater by earthing the upper plate.

Now we have already seen (p. 101) that an uncharged conductor brought near a charged one lowers the potential of the latter as a result of the opposite sign of charge which separates out on the nearside of the uncharged conductor; it is, indeed, as a result of this effect that the capacitance of the charged conductor is increased. It will be appreciated, however, that the uncharged conductor acquires an *induced potential* (by virtue of its proximity to the charged conductor) which will be of the same sign as that of the charged conductor (but of smaller magnitude). Now the existence of this induced potential reduces the extent to which the uncharged conductor lowers the potential (and increases the capacitance) of the charged one, and it is for this reason that maintaining the uncharged conductor at earth potential enhances its effect on the charged one.

(iii) If the insulated plate in the experiment just described is fixed just above the top cap of the electroscope, the latter having first been given a charge, it is found that when a sheet of dielectric (e.g. bakelite or paraffin wax) is inserted between the two plates, the divergence of the electroscope is decreased, i.e. its capacitance is further increased.

In general, we may say that the capacitance of a conductor is increased by the introduction of a dielectric between it and nearby conductors (the latter being insulated or earthed). Air itself, of course, as a dielectric, is responsible for a very slight increase in capacitance (over and above a vacuum) but this increase is so slight as to be for all practical purposes negligible.*

---

* It can be shown that the ratio of the capacitance of a conductor in a certain medium to its capacitance when surrounded by air (or strictly speaking *in vacuo*) is equal to the dielectric constant of the medium (see p. 96). For this reason dielectric constant is sometimes known as *specific inductive capacity*.

Units of Capacitance

Since
$$C = \frac{Q}{V}$$
(see p. 110),

then, if Q is unity, and V is unity, C also is unity.

Thus the capacitance of a conductor will be 1 *electrostatic unit** if 1 e.s. unit of charge placed on it changes its potential by 1 e.s. unit.

Similarly, if the practical unit of quantity (the coulomb—see p. 129) is employed, together with the practical unit of potential (the volt— see p. 129) the capacitance will be given in terms of the *practical* unit, known (after Michael Faraday) as the *farad*. Thus the capacitance of a conductor is 1 farad if its potential is changed by 1 volt when a charge of 1 coulomb is given to it. Since the farad is, in fact, a very large unit, one *millionth* of it—the *micro*-farad—is commonly used, one micro-farad being denoted by the symbol 1 μF.

CAPACITORS

It has already been noted (p. 99) that the charge on an isolated charged sphere is uniformly distributed, a fact which is illustrated diagrammatically in Fig. 45a. Suppose such a charged sphere is connected to an electroscope by a wire, and an uncharged (and preferably earthed) metal plate is brought near to one side of it (Fig. 45b). Then it is found that the charge on the sphere is no longer uniformly distributed, but has become concentrated or 'condensed' to some extent, opposite the earthed plate. At the same time the electroscope, of course, indicates a fall in the potential (i.e. an *increase* in the capacitance) of the sphere (see p. 111). It was for this reason that any arrangement introduced to increase the capacitance of a conductor came to be known as a *condenser*, although more recently this term has largely been superseded by *capacitor*.

In one of its simplest forms a capacitor may consist of two flat metal plates, separated from one another by insulating material. One of the metal plates is then connected to the conductor whose capacitance is to be increased, and the other one to earth. It is important to note at this

---

* For the more advanced student it is worth noting that the 'dimensions' of capacitance are those of *length*, and, in fact, 1 *e.s.u.* of capacitance corresponds to a capacitance of 1 *cm*.

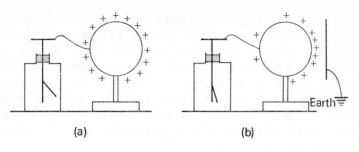

(a)   (b)

Fig. 45. The presence of an earthed metal plate near a charged sphere causes the charge to concentrate opposite the plate, and at the same time lowers the potential of the sphere.

juncture that whenever a potential difference is established between the plates of a capacitor it becomes 'charged', one plate positively, the other negatively, as shown in Fig. 46, the two charges being numerically equal though opposite in sign.

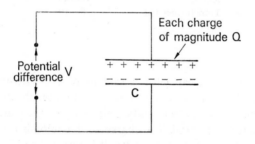

Fig. 46.

It is obvious from the discussion on capacitance (p. 110) that the action of a capacitor will be enhanced

(a) by *increasing* the surface area of its plates;
(b) by *decreasing* the distance between the plates;
(c) by introducing a solid dielectric between the plates.

It should be realized in passing that any practical form of capacitor must be so designed as to withstand the potential difference which it is required to apply between its plates, without causing a breakdown of the insulation between them.

The maximum potential difference which can be applied before breakdown occurs will depend on both the thickness of the insulating material, and on its actual composition and state (e.g. solid, liquid, or gas). So far as the thickness is concerned, it is obvious that the greater this is, the greater will be the potential difference before breakdown occurs. The effect of the material itself is to a first approximation represented by its so-called *dielectric strength*. This is an index which can be expressed, for example, as 'maximum permissible volts per mm thickness' of material. It should be realized, however, that this is a rough indication only, and that the potential difference at which breakdown occurs is not in general strictly proportional to dielectric thickness. Table V gives the dielectric strengths of some common insulating materials.

TABLE V

Material	Dielectric Strength (kV/mm)
Ebonite	30—100
Mica	80—200
Paper	3—6
Paraffin Wax	15—50
Rubber	16—40
Transformer Oil	8—10
Air	4

Capacitance

The capacitance of a capacitor is said to be 1 electrostatic unit if a charge of 1 electrostatic unit (on each plate, see above) produces a *potential difference* of 1 electrostatic unit between the plates. Similarly, the capacitance is 1 farad if a charge of 1 coulomb (on each plate) produces a potential difference of 1 volt between the plates.

A distinction should be made between the capacitance of the capacitor as a whole, and the capacitance of one of its plates considered on its own. The capacitance of one of its plates is obtained by dividing the charge on the plate *by the actual potential of the plate* in any given circumstances ($C = Q/V$). The capacitance of the whole capacitor, on the other hand, is obtained by dividing the charge (on either of its plates) by the *potential difference* between the plates. If, however, one of the plates is earthed, then the potential difference between the plates is numerically equal to the *actual* potential of the other plate, and the capacitance of the latter plate becomes numerically equal to the capacitance of the capacitor itself. It is easily seen that the formula $Q = VC$, applicable to any given *isolated conductor*, will also hold for a capacitor, V, however, denoting the *potential difference* between the plates, Q the charge (on either plate) and C the capacitance of the capacitor.

Comparison of Capacitances using a Ballistic Galvanometer

When a short pulse of electric current flows through a special type of moving coil meter (p. 156), known as a *ballistic galvanometer*, a deflection is obtained the maximum value of which is proportional to the total *charge* which has passed through the coil. Thus if two capacitors of capacitances C_1 and C_2 are charged to the same voltage V and then in turn discharged through such a ballistic galvanometer, the maximum deflections Θ_1 and Θ_2 are proportional to the charges Q_1 and Q_2 stored in the capacitors. That is

$$\frac{\Theta_1}{\Theta_2} = \frac{Q_1}{Q_2}$$

$$= \frac{Q_1}{V} \bigg/ \frac{Q_2}{V}$$

$$= \frac{C_1}{C_2}.$$

Thus this provides a simple method of comparing capacitances and if one capacitance is known, the other can be calculated.

Practical Forms of Capacitor

Capacitors have many uses, and the practical forms which they can assume are correspondingly varied: only a few representative types will therefore be considered here.

The design of a capacitor depends on the capacitance which it is desired to achieve, the potential difference which is to be applied between its plates, and, among other things, considerations of size and weight, and the atmospheric conditions in which the capacitor has to operate. Thus a 'smoothing' capacitor of relatively small capacitance, for use in the high-voltage rectifying circuit of an X-ray tube (see p. 209) will be very different from a capacitor performing a similar function in an ordinary radio set. The X-ray smoothing capacitor will be large and heavy, in spite of its low capacitance, and will incorporate a special *oil* as the dielectric, enabling it to withstand large potential differences, whilst the radio capacitor, small and compact, yet of much higher capacitance, might well consist of two long aluminium foil strips separated by thin waxed paper, wound into a tight roll and inserted into a small aluminium can for protection.

Still more compact capacitors for use in electronic equipment are made by utilizing aluminium foils, separated by paper soaked in a conducting solution known as an 'electrolyte'. Such capacitors are for this reason called *electrolytic* capacitors. Before they can be used, an extremely thin layer of aluminium oxide is formed on one of the foils by passing an electric current through the capacitor. As the oxide layer grows, the current diminishes until it reaches a minimum value for the given applied potential difference. This oxide layer constitutes the dielectric of the capacitor, separating the foil on which it is formed from the electrolyte, the latter constituting the other 'plate' of the capacitor. Since the oxide layer is very thin indeed, such capacitors have very much higher capacitances for a given overall size than the more conventional types. However, they suffer from the disadvantage of permitting the passage of an electric current, albeit a small one, during use, and usually requiring to be connected correctly with respect to polarity.

Variable capacitors, whose capacitance can be changed at will, may be constructed of two sets of parallel metal plates separated by air or thin bakelite sheets, alternate plates being joined together to form the two 'sides' of the capacitor. One set of plates can be rotated into or out of the spaces between the other set, thereby increasing or decreasing the capacitance of the capacitor. Variable capacitors of this type are used in radio sets (as tuning capacitors for example) and in other electronic equipment.

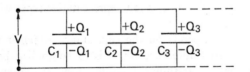 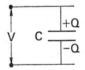

Fig. 47.

Capacitances in Parallel

Where the capacitance of an individual capacitor is not large enough for a particular purpose, an effectively larger capacitance can be obtained by connecting two or more capacitors C_1, C_2, C_3, etc. (Fig. 47) *in parallel*.

Then the capacitance C (Fig. 47) will be equivalent to C_1, C_2, C_3, etc., taken together, if the same total charge Q given either to C, or to C_1,

C_2, C_3, etc., in parallel, produces in each case the same potential difference V between the plates. Suppose the total charge Q distributes itself as shown,

C_1 acquiring an amount Q_1,
C_2 „   „   „ Q_2,
C_3 „   „   „ Q_3
etc.,

where, obviously,

$$Q_1 + Q_2 + Q_3 + \ldots = Q. \tag{1}$$

But the potential difference across each capacitance is V.

Hence, $Q_1 = VC_1$,
$Q_2 = VC_2$,
$Q_3 = VC_3$
etc.

Also, for the equivalent capacitor C, we may write

$$Q = VC.$$

Thus, substituting in Equation (1), we have

$$VC_1 + VC_2 + VC_3 + \ldots = VC,$$

whence, cancelling V throughout,

$$C_1 + C_2 + C_3 + \ldots = C.$$

That is, *the equivalent capacitance of a number of capacitors connected in parallel is equal simply to the sum of their individual capacitances.*

Capacitances in Series

Capacititors C_1, C_2, C_3, etc., connected as shown in Fig. 48 are said to be 'in series'. Then, once again, C (Fig. 48) can be considered as the *equivalent* of C_1, C_2, C_3, etc., if, when the same charge Q is imparted either to the chain of capacitors or to C considered on its own, the same overall potential difference V is produced in each case. Since the charges on the two 'sides' of a given capacitor are always numerically equal (see p. 113), it follows that when a charge Q is given to the capacitor chain shown in Fig. 48, charges separate out on its components as indicated. Then, if the potential difference across the individual capacitors C_1, C_2, C_3, etc., are denoted by V_1, V_2, V_3, etc., we may write

$$V_1 + V_2 + V_3 + \ldots = V. \tag{1}$$

But $\quad V_1 = \dfrac{Q}{C_1}, \quad V_2 = \dfrac{Q}{C_2}, \quad V_3 = \dfrac{Q}{C_3}, \quad$ etc.,

whilst for the equivalent capacitor (from Fig. 48) $V = Q/C$, where C is the equivalent capacitance. Hence, substituting in Equation (1), we have

$$\frac{Q}{C_1} + \frac{Q}{C_2} + \frac{Q}{C_3} + \ldots = \frac{Q}{C},$$

whence (cancelling Q throughout)

$$\frac{1}{C_1} + \frac{1}{C_2} + \frac{1}{C_3} + \ldots = \frac{1}{C}.$$

In words, *when capacitors are connected in series, the reciprocal of the equivalent capacitance is equal to the sum of the reciprocals of the component capacitances.*

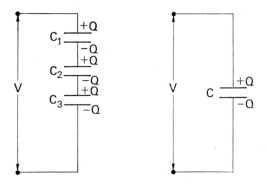

Fig. 48.

EXAMPLE

Calculate the effective capacitance of two capacitors of capacitances 8 microfarads and 12 microfarads respectively when connected in series.

If $C_1 = 8 \ \mu F$ and $C_2 = 12 \ \mu F$, then, if C is the equivalent capacitance,

$$\frac{1}{C_1} + \frac{1}{C_2} = \frac{1}{C}.$$

$$\therefore \quad \frac{1}{8} + \frac{1}{12} = \frac{1}{C},$$

$$\text{or} \quad \frac{1}{C} = \frac{5}{24},$$

whence $C = 4 \cdot 8 \ \mu F.$

EXERCISES

1. What charge is carried by a capacitor of capacitance 8 microfarads when charged to 400 volts? What would be the capacitance of the capacitor which, charged to 1000 volts, stores a charge of 20 microcoulombs?
2. Four capacitors of capacitance 1, 2, 3 and 4 microfarads respectively are connected first in series and then in parallel. Calculate the total effective capacitance in each case.
3. What is the capacitance of the capacitor which must be connected in parallel with a capacitor of 8 microfarads capacitance to provide a total capacitance of 12 microfarads? What capacitor is required in series with this same capacitor to provide a total capacitance of 2 microfarads?

THE POTENTIAL ENERGY OF A CHARGE

We have seen that work must be done to build up the charge on a conductor to its final value. Consider a conductor which is initially uncharged. Then we may imagine the total charge Q which it is proposed to place on the conductor as being built up from a large number of very small charges added successively.

The first elemental charge brought up requires no work to be done on it (just as the first layer of bricks for a brick wall can be moved along the ground and placed in position without being given any potential energy). Since the conductor now possesses a small charge, it also possesses a small potential, and work has to be done on the second elemental charge in order to place it on the conductor (just as work has to be done on the second layer of bricks in placing it on top of the first layer). In fact, the analogy between building with bricks and building up the total charge on a conductor to its final value may be pressed further. Thus the total work done in building a wall, which is a measure of the potential energy possessed by the wall when built, is obtained by multiplying the *total weight* of the wall by the *average height* (which is *half* the total height) through which the bricks have been raised,

i.e. stored (potential) energy = (half height) × (total weight).

Similarly, the energy of the charge Q on a conductor, the potential due to the charge being V, is given by the *total charge* multiplied by the *average potential* obtaining during the charging process,

i.e. energy $= \frac{1}{2}V.Q.$

It is easily shown that since $Q = VC$ the energy is also given by $\frac{1}{2}Q^2/C$, or $\frac{1}{2}CV^2$.

It is important to realize that if Q, C, and V are in e.s. units, the energy is given in *ergs*. If coulombs, farads and volts, respectively are used, the energy is given in *joules*.

THE CHARGE AND DISCHARGE OF A CAPACITOR

Suppose we wish to 'charge' a capacitor from a 'battery' of cells. The capacitor is represented by C and the battery by B (Fig. 49a). The battery has two 'terminals' T_1 and T_2, and chemical actions inside it maintain

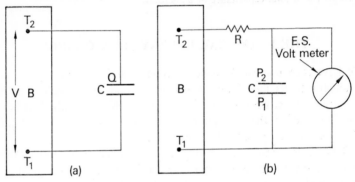

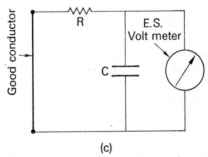

Fig. 49. Circuits for demonstrating charge and discharge of a capacitor through a high resistance.

a steady potential difference between these terminals. The two 'sides' of the capacitor are connected to the two terminals of the battery by conducting wires as shown, and the capacitor becomes 'charged'. If V is the potential difference produced by the battery, and C is the capacitance of the capacitor, then the charge Q which it acquires is given by $Q = VC$. If, after disconnecting the capacitor from the battery, an electrostatic voltmeter (see p. 108) is connected across it, the voltmeter would, of course, register a potential difference V, the charge Q acquired by the capacitor being responsible for this potential difference. If, now, a conducting path is provided between the plates of the capacitor, the reading on the voltmeter falls to zero as a result of the numerically equal and opposite charges on the two plates neutralizing each other, the capacitor being 'discharged' by an appropriate current flow along the conducting path provided between its plates.

Suppose now that the charging process is repeated, using the arrangement shown diagrammatically in Fig. 49b. One of the terminals T_1 of the battery has been connected to one of the plates P_1 of the capacitor by a good conductor (e.g. a piece of copper wire), whilst the other terminal T_2 of the battery has been connected to the other plate P_2 of the capacitor by means of a very poor conductor R, or what is usually called a *high resistance* (see p. 129). An electrostatic voltmeter is connected across the capacitor. It is then found that at the instant when the last connection is made to the battery the voltmeter does not go immediately to its final reading V, but rises, at first relatively quickly, and then more and more slowly until the final reading is attained. That is to say, the capacitor takes an appreciable time to charge when there is a high resistance connection between it and the battery. Just how long

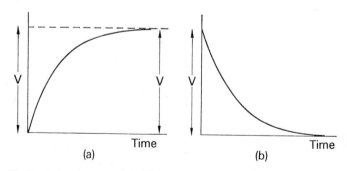

Fig. 50. Variation in potential difference between plates of a capacitor during charge and discharge through a high resistance.

9

(it may be seconds or even hours) depends, for a given capacitance, on how high the value of the resistance is: the higher this value, the longer the time taken by the capacitor to charge.

Conversely, if, after being charged, the capacitor is then *discharged* through the high resistance (Fig. 49c), it is found that the voltmeter reading does not fall immediately to zero, but decreases, at first relatively quickly and then more and more slowly until zero reading is reached. Graphically the charge and discharge of the capacitor through a high resistance may be depicted as shown in Figs. 50a and b.*

An analogy may be helpful in elucidating these charge and discharge processes and factors affecting them. Consider a water reservoir W (Fig. 51) so large that water running from it to fill the smaller vessel w will make no appreciable difference to the level of the water in the reservoir. Suppose this small vessel w is placed so that the bottom of it is level with (i.e. at the same height as) the bottom of the reservoir. This corresponds to making the first connection (T_1 to P_1, Fig. 49b) between the battery and the capacitor, for this first connection ensures that one side of the capacitor and one side of the battery are at the *same potential* (potential corresponding to height in the analogy under discussion).

Water from the reservoir is then run into the small vessel *via* a relatively narrow pipe P (corresponding to the high resistance R—for the viscosity of the water in the narrow pipe slows up the filling process). Now the vertical height (i.e. the 'head') of water in the reservoir is responsible for forcing the water through the pipe, and therefore corresponds to the potential V produced by the battery. However, as the head of water in the vessel being filled increases, the *difference* in the heads of water at either end of the pipe P diminishes steadily (just as the *potential* difference between the two ends of the resistance R diminishes steadily as the potential of the capacitor rises during the charging process). Thus the flow of water, at first relatively quick, gets steadily

---

* Actually, these graphs can be expressed in mathematical form in terms of so-called 'exponential functions'. Thus, during the charging process, the charge Q on the capacitor at any time t after the charging process begins is given by $Q = Q_0(1 - e^{-t/RC})$, where Q_0 is the *final* charge acquired by the capacitor (given by $Q_0 = VC$) and R is the value of the high resistance. During the discharging process, the charge Q *left on* the capacitor at any time t after the discharge began, is given by $Q = Q_0 e^{-t/RC}$. The product RC is known as the *time constant* of the combination of resistance and capacitance for, with increase in this product (either by increasing R or C) the time of charge or discharge of the capacitor will also increase.

slower and slower until it ceases altogether *when the level of water in the vessel w is the same as the level in the reservoir W*. This corresponds to the attainment of the full potential difference *V* between the plates of the capacitor, at which point the charging process ceases.

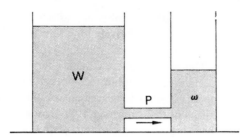

Fig. 51. Analogy illustrating the charging of a capacitor through a high resistance.

Conversely, the discharging process corresponds to the *draining* of the vessel *w* through a narrow pipe. The water is driven through the latter by the head of water in the vessel *w*, and as this head of water gets steadily less and less, the flow of water through the pipe (the 'discharge') gets slower and slower until it ceases altogether when the vessel is empty.

SOME APPLICATIONS OF ELECTROSTATIC PRINCIPLES TO RADIOLOGY

Capacitor Discharge Units

The *penetrating power* of an X-ray beam depends on the potential difference applied to the X-ray tube, which is usually stated in kilovolts (i.e. *thousands* of volts). For example, in chest radiography some 70 kilovolts (or more) will be required to give adequate penetration.

The *quantity* of X-rays employed for any particular radiograph (i.e. the 'exposure') is determined by the product of the current through the X-ray tube (usually expressed in milliamps—see p. 129) and the exposure time (usually in seconds). Thus the *exposure* is reckoned in 'milliamp-seconds' (mAs). Now the amp (see p. 129) corresponds to a current flow of 1 coulomb per second (cf. a water flow measured in *gallons* per second). The milliamp is thus a flow of 1 *milli*-coulomb (1/1000th coulomb) per second. Obviously, if the current in milliamps is multiplied by the time in seconds for which it flows, we get the total

quantity which has flowed in *millicoulombs* (cf. gallons per second ×
number of seconds, which gives quantity in gallons which has flowed).
Thus the exposure in mAs is also, numerically, the quantity of electricity
in millicoulombs which passes through the X-ray tube during the
exposure.

Now this quantity can either be obtained as a small current (a few
tens of milliamps) passing for a relatively long time (several seconds) or
as a large current (several hundreds of milliamps) for a short time (e.g. a
tenth of a second). The choice between these alternatives may be un-
important, but in certain radiographic techniques, e.g. of the chest, a
short exposure time is essential if movement of the patient is to be
'frozen'. Exposure times of the order of 1/10th second are then impera-
tive, and this, in turn, means tube currents of the order of hundreds
of milliamps.

Now the supply of such a large current to an X-ray tube normally
involves the use of heavy-duty rectifier circuits (see p. 204), and the
so-called *capacitor discharge unit* was introduced to enable these high
currents (with their accompanying short exposure times) to be attainable
without such heavy-duty supplies being necessary. The arrangement
employed is illustrated diagrammatically in Fig. 52a. The high voltage
supply circuit, instead of being connected direct across the X-ray tube,
is connected to a high-voltage capacitor *C* via the switch *S*. This switch
enables the capacitor to be charged to the full voltage of the supply,
and *then* to be disconnected from the supply and placed across the
X-ray tube, as indicated by the dotted connection. A flow of electrons
through the X-ray tube under the influence of the potential difference
between the plates and the capacitor constitutes a *current* which *discharges* the capacitor (in a small fraction of a second) and incidentally,
produces the X-ray exposure. The X-ray tube is thus seen to be equivalent to a *resistance* (*R*, Fig. 52b) through which the capacitor *C* is
discharged.

Now the X-ray tube consists essentially of two 'electrodes'—the
filament and the *anode*—sealed into an evacuated glass envelope so that
there is a small gap between them. The filament has two ends to it
which are brought out through the glass so that an electric current can
be passed through it to heat it. As a result, electrons are 'evaporated'
from the surface of the filament (see p. 201), and the number of electrons
driven off in this way depends on the filament temperature; the higher
this is, the greater the electron emission, and the greater will be the
current through the X-ray tube, under given conditions.

Thus the *temperature* of the filament (which in turn depends on the heating current passed through it) controls the *magnitude of the tube current*, and therefore the *time* taken by the capacitor to discharge, when connected across the X-ray tube. To all intents the X-ray tube behaves like a *variable* high resistance across the capacitor *C*, the magnitude of

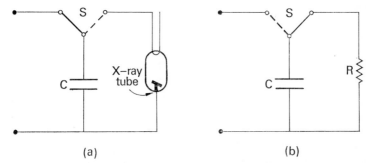

(a)   (b)

Fig. 52. The capacitor discharge unit.

the resistance (and therefore the time taken for the capacitor to discharge through it) being controllable by the temperature of the X-ray tube filament. Exposure time is thus controlled by the filament temperature, instead of by a 'timer', as employed in the more usual X-ray unit. By using a high filament temperature, a very short discharge time —and therefore exposure time—can be obtained, and for this brief time the capacitor is capable of sending a very high current (many hundreds of milliamps) through the X-ray tube. This current may, indeed, be many times the maximum current delivered by the high-voltage supply during the charging of the capacitor.

The main *dis*advantage of the arrangement can be analyzed breifly as follows. It is easily seen that if *V* is the *kilo*voltage of the supply, and *C* the capacitance of the capacitor in *micro*farads, then the equation $Q = VC$ gives the charge on the capacitor in *milli*coulombs. But we have already seen that millicoulombs are equivalent to *milliamp seconds*. Thus the exposure (in mAs) is given by the product of the *kilo*voltage, and the capacitance in *micro*farads. Now the kilovoltage is governed by the particular anatomical part to be radiographed, and it follows at once that unless the *capacitance* can be varied, the mAs also will be fixed (for a given radiographic technique). Some units have been produced in which different values of capacitance can be switched in at will, but the range of mAs (for a given kilovoltage) provided in this way is still extremely limited.

CHAPTER 7

Introduction to Current Electricity

Nowadays everyone is familiar with at least some of the properties of electric currents: for example with their ability to provide *heat* and *light*, as well as to drive vehicles, and machinery in our factories. What happens when an electric lamp is switched on? Vaguely we may say that 'electricity' flows through the lamp and that, as a result, the wire filament in the lamp is heated so much that it emits a great deal of light.

There is a useful analogy (Fig. 53) between an electric current and the water circuit of a central heating system. In the latter the fire gives heat energy to the water in the boiler, forcing it (by convection—see p. 59) to rise through the pipe connected to the top of the boiler, whence it circulates through the radiators, carrying the heat energy with it. In the radiators it loses a large part of this energy and finally flows back to the boiler.

In the electric circuit (Fig. 53b) the dynamo with its engine (or chemical action in the case of a cell) imparts kinetic energy to the electricity (i.e. to *electrons*) in the circuit, forcing a current to flow. The current in passing, for example, through lamps loses its energy and finally flows back to the dynamo or cell, round a *complete circuit*.

There are certain important implications in this analogy.

(a) The fire and boiler do not *generate* water, they merely impart heat energy to it. Similarly, the dynamo (or cell) does not generate electricity; this (in the form of electrons) is already in the circuit as a component of the material which comprises the circuit. The dynamo (or cell) merely sets this electricity in motion.

(b) Just as the heat energy conveyed by the water current is dissipated in the radiators, so the electrical energy conveyed by the electric current is dissipated in the lamps, etc., through which it is made to flow.

(c) The fire continually replenishes the energy conveyed by the water. Similarly the dynamo (or cell) replenishes the energy carried by the electric current.

The electric current must be carried through a *conductor* (p. 92), and so the wires used will, in general, be of copper. A switch represents a method of interrupting this continuous circuit (and therefore the

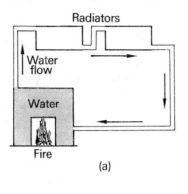

(a)

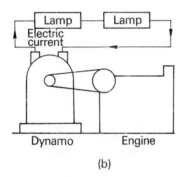

(b)

Fig. 53.

(a) In a central heating system the fire gives heat to the water and forces it to circulate through the radiators.

(b) In an electrical circuit the dynamo, driven by an engine, imparts kinetic energy to electrons in the circuit, forcing a 'current' to flow.

current) by interposing a piece of insulator (p. 92) as a break in the conducting wire. Note that the *order* in which electrical components are connected together, one after the other (i.e. in *series*), has no effect on the behaviour of the circuit.

Figure 54 shows some of the symbols used in diagrams of electrical circuits, and, as an example of the use of such symbols, Fig. 55 illustrates a circuit in which two cells in *series*, are being used to light two lamps in *parallel.* A switch is included which turns both lights on or off simultaneously, and a variable resistance (see p. 131) is also provided to control the current through (and therefore the brightness of) *one* of the lamps only.

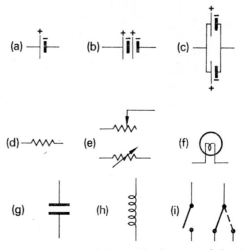

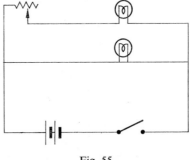

Fig. 54. Some conventional symbols used in diagrams of electrical circuits:

(a) a cell,	(b) two cells in series,	(c) two cells in parallel,
(d) a resistance,	(e) a variable resistance,	(f) a lamp,
(g) a capacitor,	(h) a coil,	

(i) an 'on-off' switch and a 'change-over' switch.

Fig. 55.

Electrical Units: Coulombs, Amperes and Volts

The *coulomb* is a unit of *electrical* quantity (or charge). The *electrostatic* unit of quantity (p. 96) is far too small for most purposes, and it was for this reason that this so-called *practical* unit was introduced, one coulomb equaling 3×10^9 electrostatic units.

The *rate of flow* of electricity is measured in practical units called *amperes* (amp). One amp is numerically a rate of flow of 1 coulomb per second, although actually this is not the way in which the ampere is defined.

Now charges (i.e. an electrical current) will flow along a conductor only when there is a difference in electrical potential between its two ends. The function of a dynamo or cell in a circuit is, therefore, to establish and *maintain* between its two ends a potential difference (*p.d.*), referred to in this case as an *electromotive force* (*emf*). The practical unit for both potential difference and electromotive force is the *volt*, and when *one coulomb* of charge is taken through a p.d. of *one volt, one joule* of work is done Correspondingly, one *erg* (10^{-7} joule) will be done in taking *one electrostatic unit* of *charge* through *one electrostatic unit* of *potential difference* (p. 106).

RESISTANCE

It follows from what has been said above that, in a circuit consisting of a number of components in series, the electromotive force generated by the cell or dynamo is engaged in maintaining a potential difference across each component. The total electromotive force is shared out in order to maintain the same current through each part of the circuit.

Ohm's Law

When the potential difference across a conductor is increased, the current which flows through it is increased too. The exact relationship is given in *Ohm's Law* which states that:

> The ratio of the potential difference applied across the ends of a conductor to the current flowing, is a constant (at constant temperature).

Thus, if a potential difference of 6 volts is found to give a current of 3 amp, it is clear from Ohm's Law that for *any* other value of potential difference, the ratio of this p.d. to the corresponding current will again be 6 : 3 or 2 : 1. The constant ratio, 2 in this case, is, therefore, characteristic of the particular conductor and is referred to as its *electrical resistance*. In fact, the resistance is *defined* as the *constant ratio* of the applied potential difference to the current flowing. If the p.d. is measured in volts and the current in amps, the resistance is said to be in *ohms*.

Factors determining the resistance of a conductor

1. In general, resistance *varies with temperature*, hence the reference to constant temperature in the statement of Ohm's Law given above. The resistance of a pure metal increases with temperature, but the resistance of carbon (which, although a non-metal, is a good conductor) falls as the temperature rises, as does that of materials incorporated into devices referred to as *thermistors.**
2. The resistance of a given wire increases with its length:
   resistance is proportional to the length of the conductor.
3. For a given length of wire, the resistance decreases as the diameter of the wire is increased:
   resistance is inversely proportional to the cross-sectional area of the conductor.
4. For wire of given dimensions (length and cross-sectional area) the resistance varies with the nature of the conducting material. The *specific resistance* (ρ) of a material is defined as the *resistance* (in ohms) of a piece of *1 cm² cross-sectional area* and *1 cm length*. The units of specific resistance are, therefore, *ohms per cm cube* (*not* per cm³).

Summarizing, then, the resistance R (ohms) of a conductor of specific resistance ρ (ohms per cm cube), length L (cm), and diameter D (cm) will be given by :

$$R = \frac{\rho \cdot L}{\pi \left(\dfrac{D}{2}\right)^2}.$$

EXAMPLE

The resistance of a length 1200 cm of wire of diameter 0·5 mm is 25 ohms. Calculate the specific resistance of the material from which the wire is made.

$$\text{Now, resistance (in ohms)} = \frac{\text{(specific resistance)} \times \text{(length in cm)}}{\text{(cross-sectional area in cm}^2\text{)}}.$$

* As resistance can be measured accurately, its variation can be used as the basis of a *temperature scale* (see p. 55) for electrical resistance thermometers. Also temperature sensors depending on the variation of resistance are used in safety and control circuits.

So, specific resistance
(ohms per cm cube)
$$= \frac{(\text{resistance}) \times (\text{area})}{\text{length}}$$

$$= \frac{25 \times \pi \times 0{\cdot}025^2}{1200}$$

$$= 41 \times 10^{-6} \text{ ohms per cm cube (approx.)}.$$

EXERCISE

1. The specific resistance of constantan wire is 49×10^{-6} ohms per cm cube. Calculate the resistance of a piece of length 1 metre and diameter 1 mm. What length of wire of *half* this diameter would have the same total resistance?

A Variable Resistance

For a given applied potential difference, the current in a circuit is proportional to its total resistance. This current can therefore be controlled by including in the circuit a *variable resistance*.

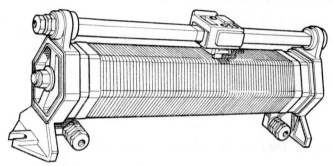

(a) A variable resistance or
rheostat.

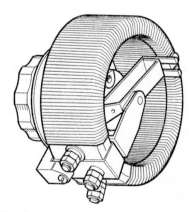

(b) A rotary type variable
resistance.

Fig. 56.

One form of variable resistance is shown in Fig. 56a. A coil of wire (having a fairly high resistance per unit length and coated with insulation to separate the turns) is wound on an insulating former. One connection to the circuit is taken to one end of the coil and the other to a *sliding contact* which can be moved along the coil, the insulation being removed from each turn at this point to provide a good connection. In this way the number of turns, that is the length and so the total resistance of the wire in the circuit can be varied.

An alternative design is shown in Fig. 56b in which the coil is wound round a strip of insulator bent into a circular arc. The sliding contact is then mounted on the end of an arm which can be *rotated* by a knob. This is a more convenient form for mounting on a control panel than the type in which the slider moves in a straight line (Fig. 56a).

Algebraical Expression for Ohm's Law

The symbols V, I and R are usually employed to denote potential difference, current and resistance respectively. Therefore, since

$$\frac{\text{potential difference (in volts)}}{\text{current (in amps)}} = \text{resistance (in ohms)},$$

we have $$\frac{V}{I} = R. \tag{1}$$

This may obviously be written in two other forms:

$$V = IR, \tag{2}$$

and $$I = \frac{V}{R}. \tag{3}$$

The resistance of a conductor can be calculated from Formula (1) above by inserting corresponding values of the potential difference, V, across the conductor (measured on a *voltmeter* in *parallel*) and the current, I, through it (measured on an *ammeter* in *series*). For such a measurement, the ammeter should, itself, have a *low* resistance, so as not to alter the current in the circuit as a whole. On the other hand, so that an appreciable fraction of the current is not by-passed through it, the voltmeter should have a *high* resistance compared with that of the conductor.

EXAMPLES

1. A p.d. of 10 volts applied across a resistance produces a current through it of 2·5 amp. Calculate the value of the resistance.

From Ohm's Law, $\dfrac{\text{p.d. (in volts)}}{\text{current (in amps)}}$ = resistance (in ohms).

Thus, in this case, resistance $= \dfrac{10}{2 \cdot 5}$

$= 4$ ohms.

2. A resistance of 200 ohms is carrying a current of 5 milliamp. Calculate the p.d. across the resistance.

From Ohm's Law (by (2) above),

p.d. (in volts) = current (in amps) × resistance (in ohms).
Thus, in this case,

$$\text{p.d.} = \frac{5}{1000} \times 200$$

$= 1$ volt.

EXERCISES

1. A torch battery of $1\frac{1}{2}$ volts emf passes a current of 0·3 amp through the bulb. Calculate the resistance of the bulb.
2. If a current of 5 amp flows through two resistances, one of 10 ohms and the other of 30 ohms, in series, calculate the p.d. across each resistance. What must be the total emf in the circuit?
3. An electric windscreen de-mister for a car has a resistance of 1·5 ohms. If the car uses a 12 volt battery calculate the current taken by the heater.

The Range of an Ammeter or Voltmeter

By the *range* of an instrument is meant the maximum reading which may be taken on it. Sometimes it is convenient to be able to alter this 'range'; for instance, an ammeter reading up to 1 amp may be required to read up to 10 amp. How can this be done?

Since the meter (of resistance R ohms, say) is required to give a full-scale deflection when a current of 10 amp is flowing in the circuit, it must be arranged that in these circumstances a current of only 1 amp is passing through the meter itself, the other 9 amp being by-passed. This can be done as shown in Fig. 57a by connecting across the meter a so-called *shunt* resistance of suitable value (S ohms, say). Since the shunt is to take 9 times the current which the meter takes, it must have 1/9 of its resistance,

$$\text{i.e.} \qquad S = \frac{R}{9}.$$

With such a shunt across the ammeter, the reading on it will need to be multiplied by 10, to give the circuit current.

Similar reasoning may be applied to show that a shunt of 1/99 of the ammeter resistance will multiply the range by 100, and so on.

It has already been pointed out (p. 132) that an ammeter, since it is placed in series with the rest of the circuit, should have as *low* a resistance as possible, whilst a voltmeter (since it is connected in parallel with a part of the circuit), should have as high a resistance as possible. An ammeter may easily be converted into a voltmeter by placing in series with it a suitable *high* resistance (Fig. 57b).

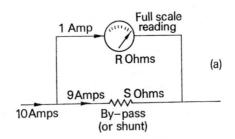

(a)

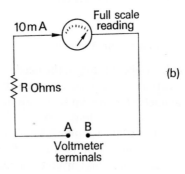

(b)

Fig. 57.

(a) Use of a *shunt* with an ammeter.

(b) Use of a milliammeter as a *voltmeter*.

EXAMPLE

Suppose a milliammeter having a range of 10 mA and a resistance of 10 ohms is required to be converted into a voltmeter, having a range of 100 volts. A resistance R ohms must be placed in series with it, such that when 100 volts are applied between the terminals A and B (Fig. 57b) a current of 10 mA will flow through the instrument.

From Ohm's Law,

voltage applied = current (in amp) × resistance (in ohms),

$$\therefore 100 = 0.01 \times (R + 10) \qquad \text{(see below)}$$
$$100 = 0.01R + 0.1,$$
$$\text{or, } R = \frac{99.9}{0.01}$$
$$= 9990 \text{ ohms.}$$

EXERCISES

1. A meter of resistance 6 ohms has a full-scale deflection of 400 microamp. What shunt resistance is required to allow the meter to give a full-scale reading of 10 milliamp?
2. The same instrument is to be used as a voltmeter to read 20 volts full-scale deflection. What series resistance would be required?

Resistances in Series

Suppose a number of resistances are connected in series as shown in Fig. 58. It seems natural to assume that, *considered as a group*, their total resistance will be equal to the sum of their individual resistances. Thus if the group shown in Fig. 58 is considered as a simple conductor, we should expect the resistance of the latter (i.e. the effective resistance between P and Q) to be

$$(8 + 3 + 5) = 16 \text{ ohms;}$$

or, in general, if R_1, R_2 and R_3 ... etc. are resistances in series, their equivalent resistance would be $(R_1 + R_2 + R_3 + ...)$. That this is actually the case may be proved formally as follows.

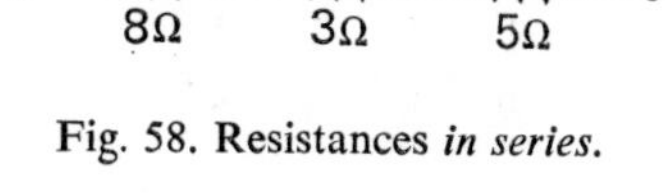

Fig. 58. Resistances *in series*.

Consider Fig. 58 again. Suppose that a potential difference of V volts applied between P and Q produces a current of I amp through the series. Then obviously, the individual resistances R_1, R_2, R_3 share the total potential difference of V volts among themselves; i.e. potential differences of V_1, V_2, V_3 exist across R_1, R_2 and R_3 respectively. From Ohm's Law, since the same current I amp flows through each, we have:

$$\text{for resistance } R_1, \quad V_1 = IR_1,$$
$$\text{for resistance } R_2, \quad V_2 = IR_2,$$
$$\text{and for resistance } R_3, \quad V_3 = IR_3.$$

Now the resistance R, to which R_1, R_2 and R_3 in series are equivalent, must obviously be of such a value that the *same* potential difference V volts applied across it, would produce the *same* current I amp through it.

Again, from Ohm's Law we have, $V = IR$.

Now, since $V = V_1 + V_2 + V_3$,

we have, by substitution, $IR = IR_1 + IR_2 + IR_3$.

Whence, dividing through by I, $R = R_1 + R_2 + R_3$, which is the expected result.

Resistances in Parallel

Any number of resistances may be connected *in parallel*, as shown in Fig. 59. It is not so easy in this case to see what their combined resistance will be. It may be observed, however, that resistances in parallel provide a number of branching paths between two points in a circuit, and that what may be termed the total *conducting power* of all the branches is obviously equal to the *sum* of the conducting powers of each separate branch. Now the conducting power of a resistance may be represented by the *inverse* or reciprocal of its resistance; for doubling the resistance will halve its conducting power, and so on. Thus the separate conducting powers of the three branches shown in Fig. 59 are 1/8, 1/3 and 1/5 respectively, and therefore, their total conducting power is (1/8 + 1/3 + 1/5). Now this must be equal to the conducting power of the resistance R, to which they are equivalent, so that

$$\frac{1}{R} = \frac{1}{8} + \frac{1}{3} + \frac{1}{5}.$$

Again we may prove this result formally, using Ohm's Law. Consider resistances R_1, R_2 and R_3 connected in parallel, and suppose that they are *together* equivalent to a resistance of R ohms. This means that if a

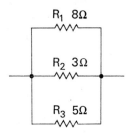

Fig. 59. Resistances *in parallel*.

potential difference of V volts across the resistances in parallel produces currents through them which total I amp, then the same potential difference of V volts must produce the same current of I amp through the resistance of R ohms, to which R_1, R_2 and R_3 in parallel are equivalent. Suppose now that the individual currents through R_1, R_2, R_3 are I_1, I_2, I_3 respectively. Then obviously

$$I_1 + I_2 + I_3 = I.$$

Now *each* of the resistances R_1, R_2, R_3 has a potential difference of V volts between its ends, and thus from Ohm's Law,

$$I_1 = \frac{V}{R_1},$$

also
$$I_2 = \frac{V}{R_2},$$

and
$$I_3 = \frac{V}{R_3}.$$

Also, since V volts between the ends of the equivalent resistance R produces a current of I amp through it,

we have
$$I = \frac{V}{R}.$$

Thus, as $I_1 + I_2 + I_3 = I,$

by substitution, we have

$$\frac{V}{R_1} + \frac{V}{R_2} + \frac{V}{R_3} = \frac{V}{R}.$$

10

Whence, dividing through by V,

$$\frac{1}{R_1} + \frac{1}{R_2} + \frac{1}{R_3} = \frac{1}{R},$$

which is the general result corresponding to the example discussed above.

Ohm's Law applied to a Complete Circuit

We know that an electric current requires a complete circuit round which to flow. Now the cell or dynamo responsible for maintaining the current must itself be regarded as a part of the circuit, the current flowing through it in the manner indicated diagrammatically in Fig. 60. Like the rest of the circuit, the cell (or dynamo) will offer some resistance to the current, and this may be called its internal resistance.

The emf generated by the cell is shared among the various circuit components (including the cell itself) in order to maintain the current through each part of the circuit, and just as we may say for an individual circuit component

$$\frac{\text{p.d.}}{\text{current}} = \text{resistance},$$

so, *for the circuit as a whole* (including the cell), we may say,

total emf operating in circuit = total of p.d.'s across components,

and $\dfrac{\text{emf operating in circuit}}{\text{circuit current}}$ = total circuit resistance.

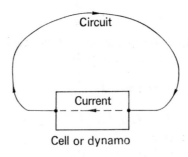

Cell or dynamo

Fig. 60. The current flows through the cell or dynamo as well as through the external circuit.

EXAMPLE

A cell of emf 1·5 volts has an internal resistance of 10 ohms. What current will flow if a resistance of 5 ohms is connected between its terminals?

Total circuit resistance = sum of resistances of circuit components
= internal resistance of cell +
external circuit resistance
= 10 + 5
= 15 ohms.

Emf of cell = 1·5 volts.

∴ For complete circuit,

$$\text{circuit current} = \frac{\text{emf of cell}}{\text{total circuit resistance}}$$

$$= \frac{1·5}{15}$$

$$= 0·1 \text{ amp.}$$

EXERCISES

1. What is the total resistance represented by three resistances of 10, 30, and 210 ohms respectively when connected in series?
2. What is the equivalent resistance of these same three resistances connected in parallel?
3. A battery of emf 12 volts has an internal resistance of 0·5 ohm and is connected to pass a current through resistances of 2·5, 6 and 9 ohms in series. What current will flow?
4. A lamp takes a current of 0·5 amp when connected across a 6 volt battery. If this lamp is to be lit by the same current from a 10 volt battery of negligible internal resistance, what resistance will be required in series with the lamp?

CHAPTER 8

The Supply and Consumption of Electrical Energy

ELECTRICAL ENERGY : ELECTROMOTIVE FORCE

An electric current can be made to do work, as, for example, when it is made to drive an electric motor or produce heat, the latter, as we have seen, being one form of energy. Thus generators of electric current such as cells or dynamos are really suppliers of energy, or rather converters of mechanical or chemical energy to 'electrical' energy. The current which they drive round the circuit acts as a *carrier* of this energy to places where it is required to be converted into heat or motion, etc.

In a steam engine the amount of energy supplied by the boiler in a given time depends not only on the amount (i.e. mass) of steam, but also on the *pressure* at which it is supplied. Similarly the amount of energy supplied by a cell or dynamo depends not only on the *quantity* of electricity (i.e. the number of coulombs), but also on what we may term the *electrical pressure* at which it is supplied. Upon the latter depends the energy imparted to each coulomb.

Now the energy possessed by an agent is measured by the amount of work it can do. Thus the *electrical pressure* (or the *electromotive force* —emf—as it is called) *of a cell or dynamo is said to be one volt if it imparts one joule of energy to every coulomb of electric charge which passes through it.*

Cells in Series or Parallel

If two cells, each (say) of emf 1 volt, are connected in series (so that each tends to send current in the same direction round a circuit), then each will give one joule of energy to a coulomb passing through it, and thus each coulomb will be supplied with *two* joules of energy, i.e. the two cells taken together have an effective emf of 2 volts. Thus argument may be used to show that in general, for cells connected in *series* (positive to negative, Fig. 61), the total emf is equal to the sum of the individual emf's.

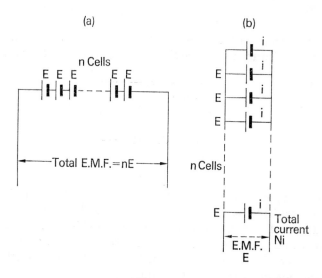

Fig. 61.

On the other hand if two cells, each of emf 1 volt, say, are connected in *parallel*, any electricity going through one does not go through the other. Thus any one coulomb receives only one joule of energy. It follows that for cells of equal emf connected in parallel (all positives and all negatives, respectively, connected together, Fig. 61b) the total emf is not increased; but for *n* cells the *total current-delivering capacity is n times greater than that of a single cell.*

WATTAGE

Suppose a battery of cells has an emf of 15 volts, and that it is delivering 3 amp to an external circuit.

Then, since 3 amp corresponds to 3 coulombs per second, and since each coulomb is given 15 joules of energy by the battery, the total energy supplied is (3×15) joules per second. Now the rate of working of 1 *joule per second* (which is a unit of *power*, see p. 47) is called (after James Watt) 1 *watt*. Thus, in the example just considered, the rate of supply of electrical energy is (3 × 15) watts. It is obvious, then, that *supply voltage* multiplied by *amps supplied* is the rate of supply of energy in watts. In short,

volts × amps = watts.

All this concerns the *supply* of electrical energy. Similar arguments may be applied to its *consumption* by any part of an electrical circuit.

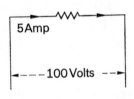

5 Amp

------ 100 Volts ------

Fig. 62.

For example, suppose an electric heating element forming part of a circuit is found to have a potential difference of 100 volts across it, and that a current of 5 amp is flowing through it (Fig. 62). In this case 5 coulombs per second pass through the heater, and each *gives up* 100 joules of energy (which is converted into heat). Thus, total rate of consumption of energy = (100 × 5) joules per sec.

= 500 watts.

Once again we may write (for each circuit component)

volts × amps = watts.

By applying Ohm's Law, this relationship can obviously also be modified to

(amps)^2 × ohms = watts,

and $\dfrac{(volts)^2}{ohms}$ = watts.

The Board of Trade Unit (the Kilowatt-Hour)

Obviously the *total* energy supplied to an electric circuit depends on two things: the *rate* at which the energy is being consumed, and the *time* for which it is consumed.

The *rate*, or power in joules per second, is given by the *wattage* of the circuit, and multiplying this by the *hours* for which the circuit is in use, we obtain the energy consumed in *watt-hours*.

In practice, to avoid large numbers, *kilo*watt-hours are used, 1 kilowatt-hour being the amount of energy consumed in 1 hour by a circuit whose *rate* of consumption is 1000 watts. The kilowatt-hour is the ordinary (Board of Trade) 'unit' by which electricity is sold.

$$\text{Since } 1000 \text{ watts} = 1000 \text{ joules per sec,}$$

$$1 \text{ kilowatt-hour} = 1000 \times 60 \times 60 \text{ joules,}$$

i.e.   1 Board of Trade unit = 3,600,000 joules,

or, since   1 joule = 10^7 ergs,

1 Board of Trade unit = $3 \cdot 6 \times 10^{13}$ ergs.

EXAMPLES

1. In a certain electric fire element the power consumption is 500 watts. What is the total energy consumption in a period of 12 hours?

Power (i.e. energy used up per sec.) = 500 watts.
∴ total energy in one hour   = 500 watt-hours.
∴ total energy in 12 hours   = 500 × 12
                               = 6000 watt-hours
                               = 6 kilowatt-hours or 'units'.

2. A resistance of 4 ohms is connected in series with a 12 volt battery, and resistances of 10 and 15 ohms in parallel. Calculate the power dissipation in each resistance.

The 10 and 15 ohm resistances connected in parallel are equivalent to a single resistance of R ohms where:

$$\frac{1}{R} = \frac{1}{10} + \frac{1}{15} \qquad \text{(p. 138).}$$

$$\therefore \qquad R = \frac{30}{5}$$

$$= 6 \text{ ohms.}$$

The total resistance of the circuit is therefore made up of the 4 ohm resistance and this 6 ohm equivalent resistance in series, making a total of (4 + 6) or 10 ohms (p. 136).

∴ from Ohm's Law for circuit, $\dfrac{\text{battery voltage}}{\text{circuit current}}$ = circuit resistance,

or $\dfrac{12}{I} = 10$, where I is the current (in amps)

∴ $I = 1 \cdot 2$ amp.

Thus the 4 ohm resistance is passing a current of 1·2 amp, and so

$$\text{power dissipation} = (\text{current})^2 \times \text{resistance (p. 142)}$$
$$= (1·2)^2 \times 4$$
$$= 5·76 \text{ watts.}$$

Considering the 6 ohm resistance, equivalent to the two resistances in parallel, we obtain from Ohm's Law:

$$\text{p.d. across resistance (in volts)} = \text{resistance (in ohms)} \times \text{current (in amps)}$$
$$= 6 \times 1·2$$
$$= 7·2 \text{ volts.}$$

A p.d. of 7·2 volts therefore exists across this pair of resistances, the circuit current of 1·2 amp dividing between them according to their relative conducting powers (p. 136).

Thus, for the 10 ohm resistance, power dissipation $= \dfrac{(\text{p.d.})^2}{\text{resistance}}$

$$= \frac{(7·2)^2}{10}$$

$$= 5·18 \text{ watts.}$$

Similarly, for the 15 ohm resistance, power dissipation $= \dfrac{(7·2)^2}{15}$

$$= 3·46 \text{ watts.}$$

THE CONVERSION OF ELECTRICAL ENERGY INTO HEAT

Consider an electric kettle fitted with an enclosed heating element, totally immersed in the water. Assume, for the moment, that *all* the electrical energy supplied to the element is given to the water as heat energy (although in practice some will be lost to the surroundings). Suppose the element has a potential difference of V volts across it, and a current of I amp through it.

Then,   wattage $= VI$.

This means that in one second VI joules of energy are converted into heat.

∴ in t seconds, energy converted $= VIt$ joules.

Now it has already been seen (p. 45) that in the transformation of energy from one form to another there is no gain or loss. The amount of energy in the second form always corresponds exactly to the amount of energy supplied in the first form, every 4·18 joules of mechanical energy being equivalent to 1 calorie of heat (p. 65).

It follows that in the above example,

$$\text{heat generated in } t \text{ seconds} = \frac{VIt}{4 \cdot 18},$$

$$= 0 \cdot 24 \; VIt \text{ calories.}$$

Alternatively, if the resistance of the heating element is known to be R ohms, then, when a current of I amp is flowing through it, since $V = IR$, we have,

$$\text{heat generated in } t \text{ sec.} = 0 \cdot 24VIt,$$
$$= 0 \cdot 24(IR)It$$
$$= 0 \cdot 24I^2Rt \text{ calories.}$$

N.B. It is obvious from the above that since no conductor has *zero* resistance, there will be *some* heat generated in all parts of a circuit, including, for instance, coils and ordinary intercomponent connections. This heat represents wasted electrical energy, and is often referred to as 'ohmic' or 'I^2R' losses. It is obvious that to minimize such losses the resistances of connecting leads must be kept as low as practicable.

EXERCISES

1. The filament of a valve operates from a 6·3 volt supply and takes a current of 0·3 amp. What is the power consumption in watts?
2. Three resistances of 5, 10 and 15 ohms respectively are connected in series with a 6 volt battery. What is the power consumption in each resistance, and the total consumption of energy in 12 hours?
3. Repeat the calculations of Ex. 2 for the case of the three resistances connected in parallel across the 6 volt supply.
4. An electric fire is labelled '500 watts, 225 volts'. Calculate the effective resistance of the element under these conditions. What would its power consumption be if this resistance were halved?
5. An electric kettle element has a power consumption of 1000 watts. Assuming for the purpose of calculation that there is no heat loss, how long will it take to boil from a temperature of 16° C if the total thermal capacity of kettle and water is 1400 cal per deg. C? (Mechanical equivalent of heat = 4·2 joules per cal.)

CHAPTER 9

The Magnetic Effects of Electric Currents

THE MAGNETIC FIELD NEAR A CONDUCTOR CARRYING A CURRENT

It was in 1819 that Oersted discovered that a conductor along which a current is flowing is surrounded by a *magnetic field*. The existence of such a field was indicated by the deflection of a compass needle near the wire when the current was switched on.

A few simple experiments suffice to indicate the general nature of this field, and the shape and direction of the lines of force.

The Magnetic Field Surrounding the Current in a Straight Conductor

A thick straight wire is passed through a card or wooden platform (Fig. 63a), on which a number of small compasses are arranged round the circumference of a circle, the centre of which lies on the wire. When a sufficiently large current is passed through the wire the compass needles are found to *point round the circle*, and since each is actually setting itself in the direction of the field in its vicinity, it follows that the *lines of force round a straight conductor carrying a current are circles, concentric with the conductor and in planes at right angles to it.*

It should be noted that if the current is reversed, the compass needles are found to point in the reverse direction round the circle.

There are a number of rules relating the direction of the current in the straight conductor to the direction of the circular lines of force round it. The simplest is perhaps Maxwell's so-called *Corkscrew Rule*, which may be stated as follows: 'If the right hand is used to turn an imaginary corkscrew (in the usual clockwise direction) so as to move the corkscrew along the wire in the direction of the current, the direction of rotation gives the direction of deflection of the north pole of the compass needle (i.e. the direction of the magnetic field due to the current).' The relative directions of current and magnetic field are therefore as shown diagrammatically in Fig. 63b.

If a sufficiently strong current is available, the experiment may be repeated using iron filings in place of the compass needles. When the platform is tapped gently, the filings are found to set themselves in circles round the conductor.

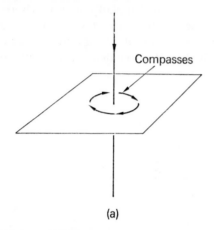

(a)   (b)

(a) Demonstration of magnetic lines of force round a straight conductor carrying a current.

(b) The relative directions of current and magnetic field.

Fig. 63.

The Magnetic Field due to the Current in a Conductor bent into the Form of a Circle

A knowledge of the nature of the magnetic field round a current flowing in a straight conductor can be employed to deduce the general configuration of the field round a circle of wire.

We may consider the circle of wire to be made up of a large number of short lengths such as *AB*, *CD*, *EF*, etc. (Fig. 64a), each of which is virtually straight. Then the current in each of these short lengths gives rise to circular lines of force, in planes which, *in each case*, are perpendicular to the short length of the conductor, as shown.

It is seen from Maxwell's Corkscrew Rule that in the vicinity of the centre of the circular conductor, all these lines of force have sensibly the same direction, being perpendicular to the plane containing the wire.

Thus, for the current direction in Fig. 64a, the lines in this region pass perpendicularly *into* the plane of paper. If the current direction were reversed, lines of force in this region would then pass perpendicularly *out* of the plane of the paper.

A more complete picture of the magnetic field associated with a current flowing in a circle of wire is easily obtainable experimentally. For example, a circular coil of wire (consisting of many turns) can be arranged half above and half below a wooden platform on which iron filings are sprinkled. When a sufficiently large current is passed through the wire and the platform is tapped gently, the filings arrange themselves in the pattern shown in Fig. 64b. It is seen that over the centre of

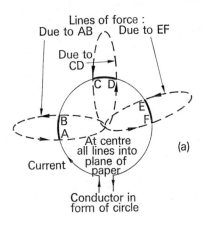

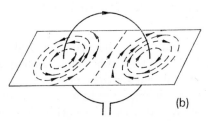

Fig. 64. Magnetic field due to current in a circular coil of wire.

the circle the lines of force are comparatively straight and, as already indicated, pass perpendicularly through the plane containing the wire. Further from the centre the lines are more curved, whilst near the wire itself the pattern includes complete loops round the wire.

The Magnetic Field due to the Current in a Solenoidal Winding

If we consider a solenoid composed of a comparatively small number of turns (as shown in Fig. 65) we can see how the magnetic field due to the current in one turn is combined with the magnetic field due to the current in neighbouring turns, and thus deduce the general nature of the field associated with the solenoid. If the current is considered to be travelling round the solenoid in the direction indicated, then the lines of force due to the first turn *ABCDE enter* that end of the solenoid, as shown. Now the lines of force inside the second turn *EFGHI* are exactly

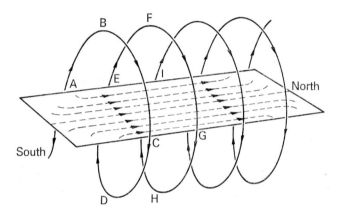

Fig. 65. Magnetic field due to the current in a solenoidal winding.

similar and combine with those from the first, in the region between the two turns, to form comparatively straight lines *linking* the two. The same argument may be applied to adjacent turns anywhere along the solenoid; and it follows that the majority of the lines of force enter at one end of the solenoid and pass along inside it for the entire length before emerging again. Outside, the lines curve round from the end from which they have emerged to enter again at the other end. It is thus seen that *the magnetic field associated with a solenoid is very similar to the magnetic field associated with an ordinary bar magnet* (p. 85). In effect, the solenoid, has, like a magnet, north and south poles, and if suspended by a fine thread to enable it to swing in a horizontal plane (the source of current being connected to it by fine flexible wires) it will set itself in the north-south direction. In addition, its poles exhibit the phenomena of attraction and repulsion of other magnetic poles, just like the poles of an ordinary magnet.

It is now obvious that it is these long straight lines of force down the inside of a solenoid which are responsible for the magnetization of a bar of magnetic material inserted in it.

ELECTROMAGNETS

A solenoid, consisting usually of many turns of insulated wire on a bobbin fitted with a soft iron core, is the simplest example of an *electromagnet*. The soft iron core becomes strongly magnetized when a

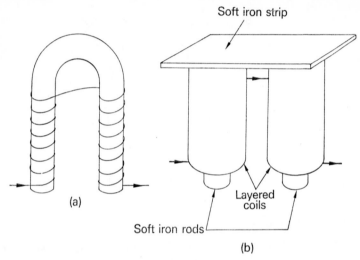

Fig. 66.

(a) A simple electromagnet.   (b) A practical electromagnet.

current is passed round the winding, and is demagnetized again when the current is switched off. Such a device (already referred to on p. 79) finds wide application in electrical equipment.

In many applications it is more convenient and efficient to employ an electromagnet of horse-shoe shape (Fig. 66a). In this case it is not usual to carry the winding round the bend. Instead, *two* windings are employed (connected in series), one on each straight portion of the core. It is important that the windings should be connected in such a manner that a south pole is obtained at one end of the core, and a north pole at the other end. The connections should, in fact, be made in such a way that if the core were straightened out, then the windings would comprise, together, an ordinary solenoidal winding. This is clearly the case if they are put on in the manner shown in Fig. 66a.

Fig. 66b shows a more convenient practical form of electromagnet of this kind, in which the core is fabricated from a flat strip of soft iron, and two cylindrical soft iron rods. Round each of these latter is a bobbin on which are wound a large number of turns of insulated wire, the two windings being connected in series in the manner just described.

The Electric Bell

The principle of the electric bell is illustrated in Fig. 67.

A is an electromagnet, opposite the poles of which is a soft iron plate *B*, mounted on a spring strip *C*. The soft iron plate carried the hammer

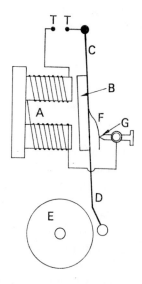

Fig. 67. The electric bell.

D. Also mounted on it is a spring contact *F* which normally touches the screw tip *G*. One end of the electromagnet winding is taken to one of the terminals *TT*, the other end being connected to the screw contact *G*. The second terminal is connected to the spring *C* (and therefore to the spring contact *F*).

It follows that when the soft iron plate (which is known as the *armature*) is at rest, there is a complete circuit between the two terminals via the electromagnet winding, the contact between *F* and *G*, and the spring *C*. Thus, if the terminals *TT* are connected to a source of emf, a current flows through the electromagnet, which consequently attracts the armature, causing the hammer to strike the gong. However, the contact between *F* and *G* is thereby broken and the current interrupted. The electromagnet in consequence ceases to attract the armature, which springs back, thus *re-making* the contact at *G*. The whole cycle of operations then starts over again. This usually takes place many times a second, causing the bell to ring so long as the connection to the source of emf is maintained.

An *electric buzzer* depends on exactly the same principle, with the practical difference that the armature is much smaller, and the spring stiffer, so that the rate of vibration is much higher than in the case of the bell. The gong is dispensed with, and the high-pitched sound is emitted by the vibrating armature itself.

Electromagnetic Relays

An electromagnetic relay is essentially an electrically operated switch, the principle of which is illustrated in Fig. 68a. Again we have an electromagnet *A*, which attracts an armature *B* when a current is passed through it. Unlike the electric bell, however, both ends of the electromagnet's winding are in this case connected direct to the terminals *tt*. Fixed to the armature is a contact *D*, which touches a contact *E* when the electro-magnet is energized. The armature (and therefore the contact) is connected to one of the terminals *TT*, the other being connected to the contact *E*. Spring *C* ensures that when the electromagnet is *not* energized the contact between *D* and *E* is broken.

The control current is connected to the terminals *tt* (Fig. 68a) of the relay, and since only a small current is required to energize the electromagnet the control circuit can be composed of comparatively fine wire, together with a simple type of switch and a low voltage source of emf. The relay itself may be designed to handle relatively heavy currents at the contacts *D* and *E* (Fig. 68a), so that the circuit to be controlled, which is connected to the terminals *TT*, may be one in which a very much larger current is flowing. Thus such a relay can be used to control the switching of a heavy-current circuit from some distant point. Only the light control circuit leads need to be run to the control switch, and the necessity for long heavy-gauge conductors is thus avoided.

The operation of a relay can, of course, be used in a similar way to *open* two contacts or, as for instance in a *telephone relay* shown in Fig. 68b, to make and break several such contacts at once or in a prescribed order.

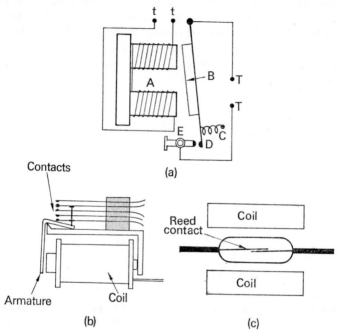

(a)

Fig. 68.

(a) The electromagnetic relay.   (b) The telephone-type relay.   (c) A reed relay.

The so-called *reed* switch is a newer form of relay which has found an increasing range of applications in recent years. It is shown diagrammatically in Fig. 68c. It comprises a pair of plated, nickel-iron alloy contact reeds, sealed into a glass envelope containing a suitable inert gas. It can be operated by means of a solenoid (into which it is inserted) or alternatively by means of a so-called proximity magnet, which may be mounted on an arm acting as the switch lever. Magnetization of the two reeds by either method causes them to be attracted to one another, closing the contacts on the ends of them. Such relays are obviously free from possible atmospheric contamination of the contacts, are fast-acting and extremely reliable.

A relay control circuit may include more than one switch in series.

In this case, the relay will not operate until all these switches have been closed, thus ensuring that contacts are not connected until *each* of a number of operations have been carried out. For example in Fig. 69, S_1 may be the control switch of an X-ray tube and S_2 the contact which is closed only when the pump, which circulates the water or oil round the cooling system to the tube, is operating. It follows that the tube cannot be switched on unless the cooling system is working, and damage to the tube by overheating is thereby avoided.

Many examples of protective circuits of this general nature will be found in any modern X-ray unit.

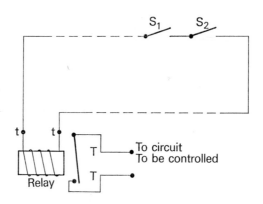

Fig. 69. The circuit connected to the terminals *TT* cannot be switched on until *both* switches S_1 and S_2 are made.

METERS TO MEASURE ELECTRIC CURRENT

Moving Iron Meters

The strength of the magnetic field produced near a conductor by the current flowing in it will obviously depend on the strength of the current itself. It follows that the intensity of this magnetic effect may be used as an indication of the current strength. Instruments using this principle are usually termed *moving iron* meters, and fall into two classes.

The *attraction type* of moving iron meter is illustrated diagrammatically in Fig. 70a. The current to be measured is passed through a solenoid S. The number of turns employed on the solenoid will depend on the magnitude of the currents which it is intended to measure with the instrument: the smaller the current the larger the number of turns required. A soft iron blade *C* is mounted on a spindle (attached to the

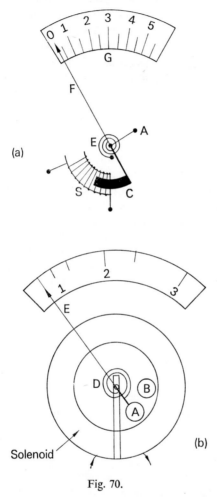

Fig. 70.

(a) The *attraction* type of moving-iron meter.
(b) The *repulsion* type of moving-iron meter.

bracket *A*), any rotation of which is opposed by the spiral hair-spring *E*, which has one end attached to the spindle and the other end to a fixed point on the frame of the instrument. The spindle also carries a pointer *F*, the end of which moves over a scale *G*.

When a current is passed, the soft iron blade *C* is attracted into the end of the solenoid, thereby turning the spindle and moving the pointer *F* round the scale. The movement ceases when the force of attraction on the soft iron blade is counterbalanced by the restoring force due to the hair-spring. Obviously, the greater the current, the greater the movement before this condition is satisfied, so that the position the pointer reaches on the scale is an indication of the strength of the current which is passing through the solenoid. The scale may be calibrated directly in amps or milliamps, according to the sensitivity of the instrument.

In the *repulsion type* of moving iron meter (Fig. 70b) there are two soft iron rods *A* and *B* inside the solenoid, which is seen end-on in the diagram. One of these (*B*) is fixed along the inner surface of the bobbin parallel to the latter's axis, whilst the other (*A*) is mounted on two arms attached to a spindle which coincides with the axis of the solenoid and also carries the pointer *E*. When a current is passed through the solenoid, both iron rods become magnetized similarly, i.e. with like poles side by side. There is therefore a force of repulsion between them, and as a result the second bar moves away from the first. The movement is again opposed by a spring *D*, and as the deflection increases with the current, the scale reading indicated by the pointer may again be calibrated to give the actual value of the current passing through the instrument.

Moving Coil Meters

A second very important type of meter is the so-called *moving coil* instrument. This makes use of what is often termed the *motor* effect, which we shall first discuss.

If a long, flexible wire connected between two fixed points is arranged to pass between the poles of a horse-shoe magnet, as shown in Fig. 71, then it is found that when a current flows through the wire it tends to move *out of*, or *further into*, the gap between the poles, according to the direction of the current (Fig. 71a and 71b respectively).

The direction of the current, the direction of the magnetic field, and the direction of the motion which ensues are *mutually at right angles*, and if Fig. 71a and 71b are examined, it will be seen that, relatively, these directions may be represented by the thumb, and first and second fingers of the *left* hand, as shown in Fig. 72. This is known as *Fleming's Left-Hand Rule.**

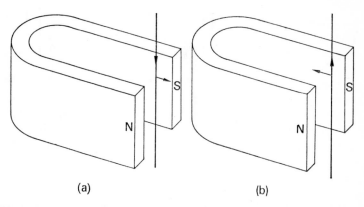

Fig. 71. A wire between the poles of a horse-shoe magnet tends to move out of or into the gap between the poles according to the direction of the current.

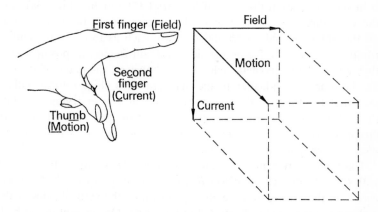

Fig. 72. Fleming's Left-Hand Rule for the direction of motion of a conductor carrying a current in a magnetic field.

* There is a corresponding *Right-Hand Rule* associated with the so-called 'dynamo' effect, to be described later (p. 168). The fact that the *left* hand is associated with the *motor* effect may be memorized by the mnemonic *L*eft-*M*otor.

Consider now, a stiff, rectangular coil of wire *ABCD* (Fig. 73) suspended between the poles of a horse-shoe magnet by two flexible wires,

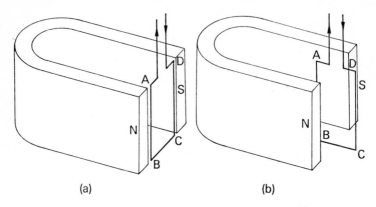

Fig. 73. A flat coil carrying a current tends to set itself with its plane at right-angles to the direction of the magnetic field.

through which a current can be passed to the coil. The application of the Left-Hand Rule to each side of the coil in turn indicates that when it is in such a position that two of its sides (*AD* and *BC*, Fig. 73a) have the same direction as the lines of the magnetic field, the forces acting on the other two sides (*AB* and *CD*) are such as to cause the coil to rotate. There is no force on the sides *AD* and *BC* in this position since they lie *along* the magnetic field. When, however, the plane of the coil has become perpendicular to the magnetic field (Fig. 73b), it will be seen that the forces acting on its sides are no longer trying to rotate the coil, but merely to increase its area, and the coil comes to rest. In fact *a flat coil in a magnetic field always tends to set itself so that its plane is perpendicular to the field.**

The forces acting may be enhanced (Fig. 74) by fitting the magnet with shaped *soft iron pole pieces B*, and supporting a *cylindrical soft iron core C* in the centre, to leave air gaps in which the vertical sides of the coil can swing freely as illustrated in the figure. On account of the high permeability of soft iron (p. 85) the magnetic lines of force are concentrated into these gaps, crossing them radially. The lines of force, the vertical sides of the coil, and the direction of motion of these sides

---

* In this position forces act on *all four* of its sides but there is no longer any turning moment on the coil.

are thus always *mutually* at right angles, provided only that the coil is
not permitted to swing through an angle sufficient to bring it out of the
gaps. This arrangement forms the basis of *moving coil meters*. The coil

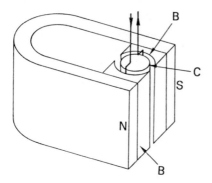

Fig. 74. Magnet fitted with soft iron pole pieces *B*, and cylindrical core *C*.

(Fig. 75) consists of a light rectangular frame around which many turns
of fine wire are wound. It is usually supported in jewelled bearings by

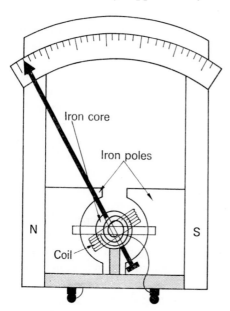

Fig. 75. The moving coil meter,

two short co-axial spindles. The coil ends are taken, one to each of the spindles, to which are attached hair-springs, which serve both to control the rotation of the coil and also to act as current leads. One of the spindles also carries the pointer. When a current is passed through the coil this rotates until it is brought to rest by the opposing hair-springs. The stronger the current the greater the movement, and, once again, the pointer reading may be arranged to show directly the value of the current flowing through the instrument. Such instruments can be made sensitive enough to give accurate measurements of currents of the order of a few micro-amps.

Some Points of Difference between Moving Iron and Moving Coil Meters

Nowadays electric power is usually supplied as *alternating current* (a.c.), that is to say, as a current which repeatedly reverses the direction in which it is flowing; in Britain, one hundred times a second.

There are practical advantages in this type of supply over a *direct current* (i.e. one where the direction of the current is always the same). Here we merely note that moving iron instruments may be used, without any modification or addition, to measure alternating current, whereas this is not the case with moving coil instruments. For, whatever the direction of the current in the attraction type of moving iron instrument the soft iron blade is always drawn *into* the end of the solenoid, whilst in the repulsion type the two iron bars are always magnetized with *like* poles adjacent and therefore repel each other. It follows that these instruments do not attempt to reverse their deflection with each reversal of the current. They thus give a definite scale reading, whether they are used to measure alternating or direct current. The inertia of the moving parts is such that the rise and fall of the current cannot be followed, with the result that an intermediate value of the current is indicated (see p. 184).

If an alternating current is passed through a moving coil instrument, the moving coil attempts to reverse its direction of deflection with each reversal of current. Since it is quite impossible for the moving coil to follow such rapid changes, no deflection at all is obtained. However, it is possible to use such a moving coil instrument in conjunction with a 'rectifier' (see p. 199), and so obtain a reading with an alternating current supply.

Moving coil instruments possess the advantage over moving iron instruments that their scales can be made strictly 'linear'; that is to say, in an instrument reading up to 10 milli-amp, for example, the size of each of the ten scale divisions will be exactly the same. (This will not in general be true of a moving iron instrument.) The reason for this is that in a moving coil instrument the strength of the magnetic field varies extremely little from point to point in the gaps between the pole pieces and the central core. Thus, to whatever point in the gap the coil moves it will always be in the same strength of magnetic field, and the same change in current will therefore always produce the same change in deflection.

On the other hand, in the attraction type of moving iron instruments described above, the non-uniformity of the magnetic field strength near the mouth of the solenoid makes it very difficult to obtain equal changes in deflection from equal changes in current over the whole range of the instrument scale. Similar remarks apply to the repulsion type of instrument, where the increase in separation of the two iron bars with increasing deflection, influences the force between them. It is to be noted, however, that there are circumstances in which this non-linearity is not objectionable and may even have advantages.

The use of shaped pole pieces and a cylindrical core in the case of a moving coil instrument produces a highly-concentrated magnetic field in the gaps in which the coil moves. Magnetic fields from nearby electrical equipment are therefore likely to be negligible in comparison, and so the reading of the instrument is unlikely to be affected by them. Moving iron instruments, on the other hand, are in general more susceptible to such interference, since the magnetic fields generated by the solenoids are much weaker than those provided by the permanent magnet incorporated in moving coil instruments.

Also, as a result of this very concentrated magnetic field, the moving coil instrument can be made much more sensitive than a moving iron instrument, but it usually suffers by being less robust in construction.

THE ELECTRIC MOTOR

The generation of *motion* by means of electric currents is one of the most important applications of electricity in everyday life. In this connection we must remember not only the obvious applications to transport, but also the innumerable uses which electrically-generated motion has in all types of machinery and scientific apparatus.

For the purpose of demonstrating the principle underlying many practical forms, a very simple electric motor can be constructed. It consists of a rectangular coil *ABCD* (Fig. 76) mounted between the poles of a horse-shoe magnet, and free to rotate about the axis *XY*. The coil

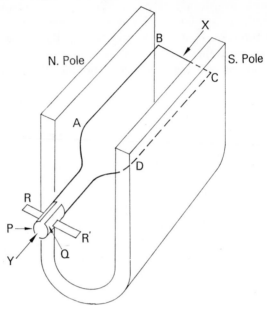

Fig. 76. The simple electric motor.

ends are attached to the two halves *PQ* of a cylindrical *commutator*. These two halves are of metal and are mounted on a cylinder of insulating material. Pressing against them, at points opposite one another in a horizontal line, are two spring contacts *RR'* (or *brushes* as they are called), by means of which the current is led into and out of the coil. Figure 77 shows three 'end-on' views of the commutator as it rotates.

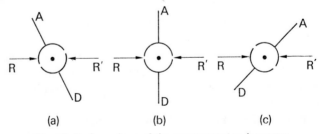

(a) (b) (c)

Fig. 77. End-on views of the commutator as it rotates.

It will be seen (Fig. 77a) that end *A* of the coil is connected to spring *R* and *D* to spring *R'*. However, after passing through the vertical position (Fig. 77b) the conditions have been reversed (Fig. 77c), *A* now being connected to spring *R'*, and end *D* to spring *R*. Thus *the commutator reverses the current direction through the coil each time the coil passes through the vertical position.* Consider Fig. 78, representing a number of successive positions of the coil, seen end-on. As we have already seen in connection with the moving coil meter (p. 158), when a current is passed, the forces on the sides of the coil will be such as to

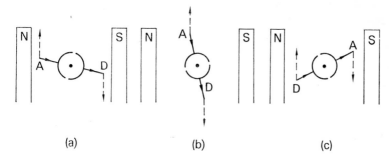

(a)   (b)   (c)

Fig. 78. Successive positions of the motor coil seen end-on.

cause the coil to rotate, if free to do so (Fig. 78a), until its plane is at right-angles to the magnetic field (Fig. 78b). Here, the forces acting on it are no longer rotational, but if its bearings are free enough, the coil will rotate past this position under its own momentum. It will be seen from the Left-Hand Rule that the reversal of the current by the commutator at this moment, results in the forces on *AB* and *CD* being such as to cause the coil to continue to rotate (Fig. 78c).

Thus, with a suitable source of current connected to *R* and *R'*, the coil will maintain a steady rotation. Such an arrangement is not capable of developing much power, and we shall now indicate briefly some of the modifications which can be made to convert this simple model into a practical electric motor.

In the first place, pole pieces may be fitted to the magnet and a soft iron cylindrical core to the coil (as in the moving coil meter), in order to concentrate the magnetic lines of force into the neighbourhood of the coil and thereby increase the turning effect or *torque* for a given current. Since the coil must make complete revolutions, however, the cylindrical core must rotate with it, and the two together form what is known as the *armature* of the motor. Instead of a single turn of wire, a number of turns are accommodated in two longitudinal slots in the core, further increasing the power developed by the motor for a given current.

Secondly, the number of slots in the armature may be increased, with a corresponding increase in the number of segments to the commutator. By means of a rather complicated connection scheme, wires can be wound into the slots, and connections brought out to the commutator segments in such a way that, as the coil rotates, the force acting on the turns of wire always aid each other in maintaining rotation. This increase in the number of commutator slots and wires has several advantages, among which are smoother torque, and elimination of a 'dead-centre' position, ensuring that the motor will be self-starting.*

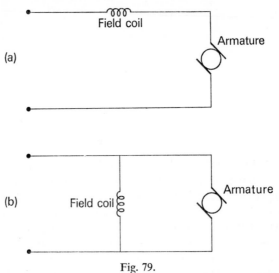

Fig. 79.

(a) A *series wound* motor.   (b) A *shunt wound* motor.

Thirdly, an *electromagnet* is generally used instead of a permanent magnet. The magnet (or 'field') coil may be in series with the armature winding (*series-wound*) as in Fig. 79a, or in parallel with it (*shunt-wound*) as in Fig. 79b. The actual choice of winding depends on the type of load characteristics required for the motor and cannot be discussed in detail here.

* For, in the simple model described in Fig. 76, if the coil should come to rest in the vertical position (after switching the current off), the coil is 'shorted out' by the commutator segments (Fig. 77) and when the current is switched on again, the motor will not start until the coil is turned slightly.

CHARGED PARTICLES IN A MAGNETIC FIELD

A stream of charged particles (e.g. negatively-charged electrons or positively-charged protons, etc.) in space constitutes a 'current' in exactly the same way as the passage of charge along a conductor. Thus, if the path of such a beam cuts at right-angles across a magnetic field, the charged particles will themselves be acted upon by a force at right-angles to both their path and the field, the direction of the force being given for positive particles by Fleming's Left-Hand Rule (p. 157). Where the particles are negatively charged, for application of the Rule they may be considered as equivalent to the flow of positive charges in the opposite direction. The magnitude of this force will be proportional to the strength of the magnetic field, the magnitude of the charge on the particle, and the speed of the particle.

Now, if a particle is acted upon by a force which is always at right-angles to its direction of motion, it will, in fact, follow a *circular* path, the radius of the latter being *inversely* proportional to the force and directly proportional to the mass of the particle.

It appears, then, that a magnetic field at right-angles to the plane in which the particles move can be used to constrain a stream of charged particles to follow a circular path, and this method is used in such instruments as the *betatron* and *cyclotron*. Further, for a given field, the *direction* of curvature of the path will indicate the sign of the charge carried by the particles, and the *radius* of curvature will give information about the magnitude of the charge, and of the energy of the particles. This principle is used to study charged particles in the *Wilson cloud chamber*, where the paths of the particles are made visible by condensed water droplets, and is also applied in the *mass spectrograph*.

CHAPTER 10

Electromagnetic Induction

THE 'DYNAMO' EFFECT

We have seen (p. 156), that a conductor carrying a current across a magnetic field tends to move in a direction at right angles both to itself and to the magnetic field. This we have called the *motor effect*.

Conversely, we might expect that if a conductor is *moved* across a magnetic field, a current will be generated in it—the *dynamo effect*. That this is actually so, can be demonstrated by the following experiment.

A straight wire, whose ends are connected to a sensitive current meter, is moved into, then out of, the jaws of a horseshoe magnet (Fig. 80a). It is found that:

(a) a current flows through the meter, its direction reversing with a reversal of the direction of movement of the wire relative to the magnetic field;

(b) the current lasts so long as the movement lasts;

(c) the *magnitude* of the current generated (as indicated by the meter deflection) depends on the *rate* of movement of the conductor across the field, the faster the movement the greater the current.

In the *motor* effect the relative directions of current, magnetic field, and movement generated are given by Fleming's *Left*-Hand Rule (p. 157). In the *dynamo* effect, it can be shown that a similar rule applies, making use of the *right* hand, however. This rule can be deduced from the following considerations.

Suppose a current is passed *through* the wire as shown in Fig. 80b. Then, if free to do so, the wire will move in the direction indicated (Fleming's Left-Hand Rule). But we know now that *as a result of this movement*, a current will be induced in the wire, and that this current will persist so long as the motion persists. Now this 'induced' current will either aid or oppose the original current. If it aided it then the total current would be increased, bringing about an increased motion, which in turn would produce a further increase in current, and so on. This process would represent energy for nothing, which we know is contrary to experience.

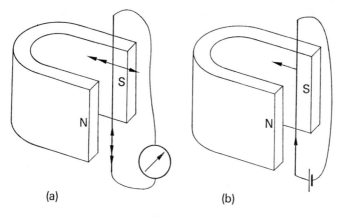

Fig. 80.

(a) A current is induced in a conductor when it is moved into or out of the gap between the poles of a horseshoe magnet.

(b) If a current is passed through the wire it will tend to move in the direction indicated.

It follows that the induced current must *oppose* the original current responsible for the motion. In more general terms this becomes *Lenz's Law*: *the direction of the induced current is always such as to oppose the cause producing it* (e.g. motion, or in the above case, the original current responsible for the motion).

Hence, for motion into the jaws of the magnet shown in Fig. 80a, the induced current will be downwards, and *vice versa* if the movement is reversed. This can be presented by a *Right*-Hand Rule, in which the *thumb* again stands for *motion*, the *forefinger* for the *field*, and the *second* finger for the direction of the resultant induced *current* (Fig. 81).

It is very important to realize that even when a complete circuit is not provided for the induced current to flow round, there will still be an *electromotive force* induced, as, for example, between the ends of the wire in Fig. 80a, even when no meter is connected across it. It is in fact this induced emf which *causes* the observed current when a complete conducting path is provided.

As we have already seen, the magnitude of the induced current (or more correctly the magnitude of the induced emf) depends, among other things, on the *rate of movement* of the conductor across the magnetic field. Actually it can be shown that the induced emf is directly proportional to the rate at which lines of force are cut by the conductor (often referred to as *Faraday's Law of Electromagnetic Induction*).

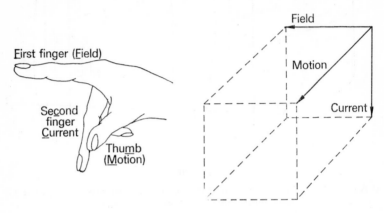

Fig. 81. The Right-Hand Rule for the direction of the induced current in a conductor moving in a magnetic field.

It is helpful at this point to observe that the action of the conductor in cutting lines of force is much the same as the action of the cutters of a lawn mower in cutting blades of grass: the faster the mower moves across the lawn the greater the number of blades of grass cut per second; also the wider the cutters the more grass is cut for a given rate of movement. Similarly, for the conductor, the rate of cutting of lines of force (i.e. number cut per second) depends not only on the conductor's *rate of movement* but also on its *length*, doubling the length doubling the rate of cutting, and so on. It is to be noted, too, that just as in order to cut the grass the cutter must move at right angles to the grass blades, so, in order to generate an emf, the conductor must move *across* lines of force: no amount of movement, however fast, along the lines of force will generate a current. It follows that if a conductor is moving at a given speed directly *across* a magnetic field (giving maximum cutting rate of lines of force) the induced emf will be at a maximum, and that if the *direction* of movement is gradually changed (without change of speed) until it is along the magnetic field, the induced emf will fall steadily to zero.

The Alternator and D.C. Dynamo

Consider again the case of a simple rectangular coil *ABCD* rotating about an axis *XY* between the poles of a magnet, as shown in Fig. 82.

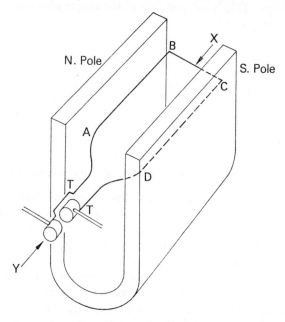

Fig. 82. The simple alternator.

Then, as the coil rotates, it will pass through the positions shown (seen from the end of the coil) in Fig. 83. Imagine the sides *AB* and *CD* to correspond to the rotating cutters of the lawn mower. At the moment represented by Fig. 83a they are cutting straight across the field (*AB* up and *CD* down, say), and the induced emf (which appears between the ends *TT* of the coil) will be at a maximum. In position Fig. 83b the motion of *AB* and *CD* is no longer directly across the lines of force, and in consequence the emf will have fallen in value. At the position shown in Fig. 83c, *AB* and *CD* are momentarily travelling directly *along* the lines of force, and the emf is at this instant zero. At Fig. 83d it has begun to increase again, *but acts in the opposite direction* (since *AB* is now travelling *downwards* and *CD* *upwards*) until it reaches a maximum at Fig. 83e. After this it falls again to zero (Fig. 83f), and rises to a maximum again in the original direction (Fig. 83g). The whole cycle is then repeated as the coil continues to rotate. Such an induced emf is said to be an *alternating* one, and may be applied to an external circuit simply by taking the coil ends to a pair of continuous *slip rings*, as shown in Fig. 82, against each of which presses a *brush* contact, connected to the external circuit. This is the principle of the simple *alternator*, or alternating current generator.

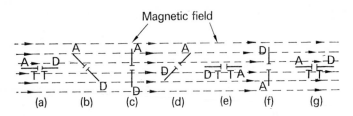

Fig. 83. An end on view of coil rotating in the magnetic field.

We may note (see p. 174) that a 'crest' together with a 'trough' constitutes what is known as one complete *cycle* of the alternating emf, the number of complete cycles generated in one second being known as the *frequency*. In Britain alternating current is supplied by the mains at 50 cycles per second, but in the USA 60 cycles per second is usual.

If we wish to prevent actual reversals of current in the circuit connected to the simple generator described above, a two-segment commutator (as in the case of the simple motor, Fig. 76) can be fitted. In this way, at the instant when the emf at the coil ends (*TT*) is reversed (Fig. 83c and f), the connections to the external circuit are also reversed, thus preventing reversals of current at the circuit itself. Such a generator is known as a *d.c. dynamo*.

It must be realized that, obtained in this way, the current, although direct, is by no means *steady* in value, fluctuating as it does between a maximum and zero.

As in the case of the electric motor, considerable modifications are necessary to the simple arrangement described, to obtain a machine suitable for practical purposes. These modifications cannot be considered in detail, but tend to follow the same general lines as those applicable to the electric motor (p. 161):

(a) The number of turns in the rotating coil can be increased.

(b) The rotating coil can be fitted with a soft iron core.

(c) An electromagnet can be used to produce the field in which the armature rotates. (The current *generated* by the dynamo may be used for energizing the magnet, in which case a slight residual magnetic field is necessary to start the action. This is usually present in the form of weak permanent magnetization of the magnetic core.)

(d) The armature winding can be made more complex than that corresponding to a flat coil, an increase in the number of segments on the commutator then being necessary. An important result of modifying the armature winding in this way is the production of a steadier direct current, with a reduction in the fluctuations or 'ripple'.

SELF AND MUTUAL INDUCTANCE

Suppose a magnet is moved towards a flat coil, as shown in Fig. 84a. Then it is clear that the nearer the magnet gets to the coil, the greater will be the number of lines of force passing through the area surrounded by the coil. Each line, as it becomes linked with the coil, is obviously

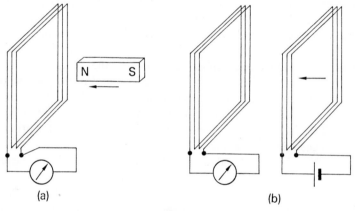

(a)   (b)

Fig. 84.

(a) If a magnet is moved towards a flat coil, an emf is induced in the coil whilst the magnet is in motion.

(b) If a coil carrying a current is moved towards a second coil, an emf is induced in this second coil whilst the first is in motion.

cut by the latter in the process. Thus an emf is induced in the coil, whose magnitude will be proportional to the *rate* of change of the number of lines of force linked with the coil at that instant. When the number is *increasing* (magnet approaching) the induced emf will act in one direction. When the number is decreasing (magnet receding) it will act in the opposite direction. It will also reverse when the other pole of the magnet is used.

The direction of the induced current can be obtained from Lenz's Law if we remember that when a current flows in a coil, the magnetic field which it sets up is such that one face of the coil may be considered of north polarity, and the other of south polarity. Lenz's Law then indicates that the polarity of the face nearer the magnet's pole must be the *same* as the latter when the magnet is being moved *towards* the coil (thus repelling it), and *opposite* to it when the magnet is moved away (thus attracting it). In each case the induced current attempts to prevent the relative movement of magnet and coil.

Obviously the magnet can be replaced by another coil in which a current is flowing (Fig. 84b). Then, instead of moving the coil, as was done with the magnet, the magnitude of the current in this coil (the *primary*) can be varied. This will alter the magnetic field linked with the second coil (the *secondary*), in which there will be an induced emf *so long as the current in the first coil is varying*. These two coils are said to have a *mutual inductance*. The more *rapidly* the current in the primary varies, the larger will be the induced emf in the secondary. If the secondary circuit is complete, an induced *current* will flow in a direction to produce a magnetic field of its own opposing the change due to the other coil. Thus the induced emf will be in one direction whilst the primary current is rising, and reversed when it is falling. The *mutual inductance* of the two coils (or circuits) is said to be *one henry* (plural *henries*) if the induced emf in the secondary is *one volt* when the primary current is changing at the rate of *one amp per second*.

Even with a *single* coil, induction effects will be observed. If a current is flowing in this coil, there is a corresponding magnetic field. If the current varies, this magnetic field linked with the circuit also varies and so an induced emf is produced to oppose the change. If the current is increasing, the induced emf will oppose the rise; if the current is falling the emf will try to maintain it. This is due to the *self-inductance* of the coil (or circuit) and, similarly, the self inductance is said to be *one henry* if the induced *back* emf is *one volt* when the current is varying at the rate of *one amp per second*.

These induced emf's, which result from either the self or mutual inductance of the circuits, only occur when the currents are *varying*, when they act to oppose the changes in current. Obviously they never quite succeed, for if the current change was completely overcome, there would be no induced emf. With *direct* (i.e. constant) currents the effects of inductance will be observed only when current is switched on or off; the steady current, as determined by the resistance of the circuit and Ohm's Law, is not affected. However, with an *alternating* current (see p. 174) which is varying continuously, the inductance will lead to an induced emf which is also varying. Thus in order to be able to calculate the net emf in the circuit, and so the current flowing, both the *resistance* and the *inductance* must be known. Also the high mutual inductance of two coils wound on a common core forms the basis of the operation of the alternating current *transformer*. These two subjects are discussed in the next chapter.

CHAPTER 11

Alternating Currents

There are a number of practical advantages, from the point of view of generation, transmission and utilization of electrical energy, in the use of *alternating* voltages and currents. These are supplies which are reversing direction many times per second in contrast to the *direct*, constant, supply from a battery. In this case the voltage (or current) varies rapidly with time from zero to some peak value, down to zero again, to the same peak value with the reverse polarity and back to zero (Fig. 85). The number of such complete *cycles* of variation completed in one second is referred to as the *frequency* of the supply, this being normally 50 cycles per sec in Britain, but 60 cycles per sec in some other countries (e.g. in the USA). Both the voltage and current will show the same frequency, the usual form of the variation being as shown in Fig. 85, a curve known mathematically as a *sine wave** (or a *sinusoidal* wave form).

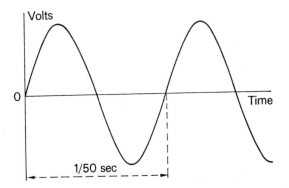

Fig. 85. The voltage goes through one complete cycle every 1/50th sec.

* See 'Mathematics for Radiographers', p. 118.

THE ALTERNATING CURRENT TRANSFORMER

If two coils are wound on the same iron ring (Fig. 86a) the lines of force from the first coil (the primary) will be concentrated in the iron and pass through the second coil (the secondary). Then these two coils will have a very high *mutual inductance* (p. 172). If a direct current were to be applied to the primary coil, the magnetic field would change only when this current was switched on or off. Thus there would be a pulse of induced emf in the secondary circuit when the primary current was switched, but there would be no induced emf whilst the primary current

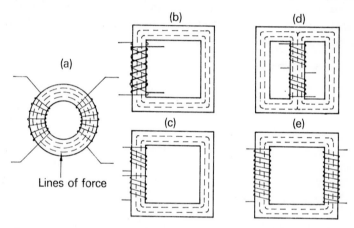

Fig. 86. Core and winding arrangements for alternating current transformers.

was steady. However, if an *alternating* current flows in the primary coil, the associated magnetic field in the iron ring will be changing continuously (except, momentarily at the peak and trough of the cycle). This varying field will be linked with the secondary coil and so (as predicted by Faraday's First Law of Electromagnetic Induction, p. 168) an emf (which is also continuously changing) will be induced in this coil. As a result, an alternating current will flow in the secondary circuit if this is completed. This arrangement is then referred to as an alternating current *transformer*. Other shapes of iron core are generally used in practice, for example, a *rectangular* core may be employed with primary and secondary wound one on top of the other or side by side on the same 'limb' (Fig. 86b and c), with the coils on opposite limbs (Fig. 86e) or side by side on a central limb (Fig. 86d).

It can be shown that the *wave form* of the induced emf is exactly the same as that of the alternating voltage applied to the primary coil, that is the two voltages will have the same *frequency* of variation (p. 174). Their relative magnitudes will depend on the mutual inductance between the coils. For a given primary coil and current, the magnetic flux linked with the secondary circuit will increase in proportion to the number of turns on the secondary coil. Therefore, with more turns on the secondary coil, the rate of variation of the flux linkage will be higher, and so (as predicted by Faraday's Second Law of Electromagnetic Induction, p. 168), the peak value of the induced secondary voltage will be higher. Now the maximum magnetic flux in the core is related to the peak primary current, which, in turn, depends on the peak value of the applied alternating voltage and the number of turns on the primary coil (determining its *inductance*).

It can be shown that:

$$\frac{\text{peak voltage across secondary coil}}{\text{peak voltage across primary coil}} = \frac{\text{number of turns on secondary coil}}{\text{number of turns on primary coil}}$$

However, it should be noted that this relationship applies for the so-called *open-circuit* secondary voltage, that is, the induced voltage with no secondary circuit connected and so no secondary current flowing. When secondary current does flow, the peak secondary voltage will be reduced as a result of energy losses in the transformer (see p. 179).

From the above formula it is clear that the transformer may be used for transforming a small peak voltage to a larger one by arranging that the number of turns on the secondary is greater than the number of turns on the primary (a *step-up* transformer). Conversely, the peak value of an alternating voltage will be reduced if the number of turns on the secondary coil is less than on the primary (a *step-down* transformer). Many transformers, in fact, have several secondary coils so that a number of different circuits can be supplied simultaneously with a range of voltages and currents.

Although it is usual to consider a transformer as having *two* coils wound on the same core, there is strictly no reason for these coils to be independent. Thus, in an *auto-transformer* there is only a single coil, tapped as shown in Fig. 87.

The whole coil constitutes one winding and the tapped portion of the same coil forms the other winding. According to which is used as the primary (the whole or the part winding), the auto-transformer will provide either a step-down or step-up in voltage. As the currents oppose each other in the common part of the coil, resistance losses (see p. 178)

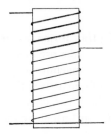

Fig. 87. The auto-transformer.

are reduced and thinner wire can be used than in a normal transformer of the same rating. The auto-transformer is therefore cheaper and less bulky. For a voltage ratio not very different from unity there is no objection to this design, but if the secondary circuit as a whole is at a very different potential from that of the primary (e.g. when supplying the filament of an X-ray tube, see p. 205) two separate, well-insulated coils must be used as in a normal transformer. However, it is very easy to arrange for multiple tappings to the single coil of an auto-transformer. These can then be used for variation (in small steps over a limited range) of the voltage applied to the main X-ray high tension transformer (kV control) or to provide a means of compensation for small variations in the mains supply (a mains compensator).

It will be clear from the above discussion that the transformer is a very useful device. In fact, it is the ease with which the magnitude of a voltage can be changed (either up or down) by means of a transformer that offers one of the great advantages of an alternating supply. This is obviously useful in connection with radiological equipment where high voltages (e.g. 200 kVp) are required across the X-ray tube, but low voltage (e.g. 6 volts) supplies are needed for the valve and tube filaments (p. 202). Transformers are also useful in connection with the transmission of electricity over long distances. The cost of overhead cables depends mainly on the actual *amount* of material in the conductors. If a high voltage can be used the same total power can be carried at lower current, when cables of smaller diameter (and so higher resistance) can be utilized without excessive energy loss. Thus the supply is transformed to very high voltages for transmission (e.g. 33 kV, 132 kV or 275 kV on the 'grid' in Britain) and then reduced to lower voltages again (e.g. 440, 230 or 110 volts) for supply to the individual users.

Power in a Transformer

It is convenient to regard a transformer as an electrical *machine* without moving parts. We may then make use of some of the ideas discussed in Chapter 3 in connection with machines in general. If the transformer is *perfect*, the energy got out of it in a given time will be equal to the energy supplied to it. If we consider one second, the energy may be measured in watts and for a perfect transformer we may write:

primary wattage = secondary wattage,

i.e. primary voltage × primary current (in amps) =

secondary voltage × secondary current (in amps),

$$\text{or } \frac{\text{secondary voltage}}{\text{primary voltage}} = \frac{\text{primary current}}{\text{secondary current}}.$$

Thus, a step-*up* in voltage implies a step-*down* in current and *vice-versa*: an increase in voltage is, so to speak, paid for by a decrease in current and an increase in current is only obtained at the expense of a decrease in voltage. Where there are several secondary circuits we must, of course, write for the perfect transformer:

primary wattage = *total* wattage of all secondary circuits.

Transformer Losses

In practice, like all other machines, the transformer will not be perfect, and the energy obtained from it in a given time will be *less* than the energy supplied to it for the reason that there are losses of energy in the transformer itself, analogous to the frictional losses in an ordinary machine. Some of these energy losses are associated with the windings (which are of copper wire), and are referred to as *copper* losses, and some with the (iron) core, therefore known as *iron* losses. Copper losses arise from the fact that the windings have a finite (and not zero, even though usually small) resistance, and so they are *heated* to some extent by the current flowing through them (see p. 144). The greater the resistance of a winding, the greater will be the heat generated in it for a given current through it, i.e. the greater will be the copper losses. Thus wire as thick as is practicable must be used in order to minimize such losses. Iron losses are considered in a later section (p. 181).

As with other machines (p. 49) we refer to the *efficiency* of the transformer as being given by the ratio of power output to power input, expressed as a percentage. That is,

$$\text{efficiency} = \left(\frac{\text{power output}}{\text{power input}} \times 100 \right) \%.$$

As the losses will increase with the magnitude of the current drawn from the transformer, the efficiency will fall. For a given primary voltage and turns ratio the secondary voltage will fall as the secondary current increases, being maximum on 'open circuit', i.e. when no circuit is connected to the secondary coil. It is desirable, in practice, that the fall of secondary voltage between 'open circuit' and the normal load secondary current should not be too great, and, in fact, this fall is related to the efficiency of the transformer. The effect is measured by what is termed the *regulation* of the transformer, which is expressed as a percentage and defined as

$$\left(\frac{\text{open circuit secondary volts} - \text{secondary volts on load}}{\text{open circuit secondary volts}} \times 100 \right) \%.$$

For X-ray sets this regulation is expected to be not more than about 10 per cent.

It will now be seen that for a given primary voltage the secondary voltage depends on the step-up ratio of the transformer and to some small extent on the load current drawn from the secondary coil. For given load conditions it is possible to calibrate a meter reading the primary voltage so that it indicates the *secondary* voltage obtained, and this procedure is fairly generally adopted in X-ray equipment. An alternating current voltmeter (frequently a moving iron meter) is connected across the primary of the transformer, and is calibrated at the factory to read *peak* transformer *secondary* voltage under specified load conditions.

EXAMPLES

1. A 6 volt lamp operated at 48 watts from a transformer with 240 volt input, has an efficiency under these conditions of 90%. Calculate the primary and secondary currents of the transformer.

Let the primary and secondary currents for the transformer be I_p and I_s amp respectively.

$$\text{Then, input power} = 240 \times I_p \text{ watts.}$$

$$\therefore \text{ output power} = (\text{input power}) \times (\text{efficiency})$$

$$= 240 I_p \times \frac{90}{100}$$

$$= 216 \, . \, I_p \text{ watts.}$$

But, output power = 48 watts.

$$\therefore \text{ primary current, } I_p = \frac{48}{216}$$

$$= 0 \cdot 22 \text{ amp.}$$

Also, output power = (secondary current) × (secondary volts)

$$\therefore 48 = I_s \times 6$$

$$\text{or, secondary current } I_s = \frac{48}{6}$$

$$= 8 \text{ amp.}$$

2. Calculate the step-up turns ratio required by a transformer which is to provide a secondary voltage of 100 kV from a primary supply of 230 volts, given that the transformer regulation under these conditions is 10%.

$$\text{Regulation} = \frac{\text{fall in secondary volts on load}}{\text{open circuit secondary volts}} \times 100\%$$

$$= 10\% \text{ in this case.}$$

$$\therefore \text{ fall in sec. volts on load} = \left(\frac{10}{100}\right) \times (\text{open circuit volts}).$$

$$\text{Thus, secondary volts on load} = \frac{9}{10} \, (\text{open circuit volts})$$

$$= 100{,}000 \text{ volts, in this case.}$$

$$\text{i.e. open circuit sec. volts} = \frac{10}{9} \times 100{,}000$$

$$= 110{,}000 \text{ volts approx.}$$

$$\text{Then, step-up turns ratio} = \frac{\text{open circuit secondary volts}}{\text{primary volts}}$$

$$= \frac{110{,}000}{230}$$

$$= 480 \text{ approx.}$$

EXERCISES

1. The primary coil of a transformer is fed from a 250 volt alternating supply. The turns ratio corresponds to a step-up of 400/1. Calculate the 'open circuit' secondary voltage.
2. For a secondary current of 5 milliamp the regulation of the transformer referred to in Ex. 1 is 9%. Calculate the secondary voltage, and hence the transformer efficiency, under these load conditions, if the primary current is 2·05 amp.
3. A transformer primary is fed from a 225 volt alternating supply, and provides a secondary voltage of 50 kV at a current of 1·8 mA. Calculate the primary current if the efficiency of the transformer is 95%.

Eddy Currents

Consider again the iron core of the transformer, and imagine it to consist of a number of cylinders each fitting into the other. (Fig. 88). It is then clear that some of the lines of force running along the core from one end to the other will be *linked* with these imaginary cylinders (each of which may be regarded as a single continuous 'turn' of a very wide metal strip). Induced currents will therefore flow round these cylinders whenever the magnetic field changes (i.e. whenever the primary current changes), and as the resistance is low, the currents will be large. Such unwanted induced currents, appearing incidentally in the metal parts of electrical apparatus in which there are changing magnetic fields, are usually referred to as *eddy currents*. In consequence of them the metal parts in which they flow become heated to some extent, a process which represents a waste of energy. In the majority of cases the metal concerned is an iron core, and this wasted energy is then included (together with hysteresis losses—see p. 87) in what were referred to as 'iron losses' (p. 178).

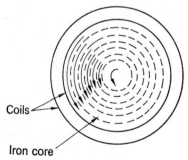

Coils

Iron core

Fig. 88. The production of eddy currents in the core of a transformer.

According to Lenz's Law, in the case of the core of the transformer the direction of the current round our imaginary cylinders will be such as to oppose the change (i.e. the growth or decay of the magnetic field) producing it. It follows that the eddy currents circulate round the core in the opposite direction to that in which the primary current circulates whilst the latter is *growing*, reversing direction as the primary current falls. In an exactly similar manner eddy currents are set up in the core of any inductance.

Eddy currents are also set up in the iron armature core of an electric motor. In this case it is the *motion* of the iron core in the magnetic field which gives rise to the currents. Their general direction will be *across* the magnetic field, and they will be at a maximum in a plane parallel to the field and containing the axis of rotation.

If the eddy current path within the metal is considered as a closed circuit of resistance R in which an emf E is induced, the energy loss, which will appear as heat, is given from Ohm's Law as E^2/R. E depends only on the variation in the magnetic linkage which occurs, and so, to reduce the eddy current energy loss, it is necessary to increase R, the resistance of the eddy current path in the metal.

For two coils linked by a single straight iron rod this could be done by making this core from a bundle of iron wires so as to insulate each one from its neighbour. The resistance to the eddy currents flowing from one wire to another would then be so high that the energy loss would be greatly reduced. Eddy currents could of course still circulate within each wire with a low resistance path, but as the wires would be of small diameter the number of magnetic lines of force enclosed in this path would be small, and so the induced emf and the energy loss involved would also be small.

For similar reasons transformer cores, and armature cores of electric motors and dynamos, are in practice, built up from thin varnished or oxide-coated *laminations* of soft iron sheet, stamped out to the right shape. These are arranged so that the path of the induced eddy currents is from lamination to lamination, and is therefore of very high resistance, thus again minimizing the energy loss involved.

Eddy currents do find practical application in certain instances. For example, the coils of moving coil meters are often wound on metal formers (from which they are, of course, insulated) in which eddy currents will be induced when the coil rotates in the magnetic field. The direction of these eddy currents will be such as to set up additional forces which oppose the motion of the coil. It is important to note that these additional forces will not play any part in determining the final position taken up by the coil, since they vanish when the motion ceases. Their effect is to *damp down* the movement of the coil and to make it relatively 'sluggish'. In particular, it can be arranged that when the instrument is in use the coil does not oscillate about its final position before coming to rest—it swings straight up to this position and stops. The movement is then said to be 'dead-beat', and such an instrument is quicker and easier to use than one which does not have this arrangement incorporated.

Another important application is in *eddy-current heaters*. These find considerable use in the manufacture of radio valves and X-ray tubes, in which metal parts are to be included in a highly-evacuated glass envelope. Gas is trapped ('absorbed') within the metal surfaces and if released subsequent to the envelope being sealed this gas will spoil the high vacuum required for the operation of the tube. Therefore, during the pumping process it is necessary to heat these metal parts to drive off the gas, without at the same time melting the glass envelope. This is done by placing the tube within a solenoid carrying an alternating current of very high frequency (several million alternations a second). The eddy currents induced in the metal parts inside the glass are then sufficient to produce red heat in the metal parts, whilst the glass, as a non-conductor, is unaffected.

VOLTAGE-CURRENT RELATIONSHIPS IN AN ALTERNATING CURRENT CIRCUIT

Circuit Containing Resistance Only

If an alternating supply is connected to a resistance (as shown diagrammatically in Fig. 89a) the current I *at any instant* will be given by Ohm's Law applied to the resistance R and the corresponding (instantaneous) value V of the potential difference. Thus the current will vary cyclically in step (or *in phase* as it is called) with the applied potential difference, with a constant ratio (numerically equal to the resistance) between their values (curves V and I in Fig. 89b, where, of course, the ratio of the heights of the peaks V_0 and I_0 is also determined by the resistance).

Now it has been shown (p. 142) that the power dissipation in watts in a resistance (or what amounts to the same thing: the rate of production of heat in the resistance) is given by the product VI, where V is the potential difference in volts and I the current in amps. From Ohm's

Law this equals I^2R, where R is the resistance in ohms. Thus the power dissipation at any instant is proportional to I^2, and the variation of I^2 with time is also shown in Fig. 89b. It is to be noted that this always remains positive, as the sign of I^2 is the same for $(-I)^2$ and $(+I)^2$. If the *average* value of I^2 during one complete cycle is denoted by $\overline{I^2}$, then a constant current I_{eff} (equal to the square root of this average of I^2) would give the same energy dissipation in the time of one cycle as the given alternating current. I_{eff} is therefore the *equivalent* direct current from the point of view of heat production, and is known as the *effective* or *root mean square* current (i.e. the *square root* of the *mean* value—over one cycle—of the *current squared*). The root mean square voltage V_{eff} may be defined in an exactly similar fashion.

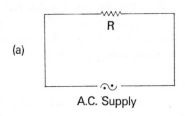

(a)

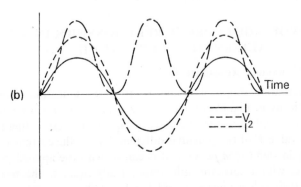

(b)

Fig. 89.
(a) An alternating current circuit containing resistance only.
(b) Alternating voltage V and current I in this circuit.

For a sine wave variation the average value of I^2 over one cycle is in fact half the peak value of I^2, i.e. $I_0^2/2$, where I_0 is the value of the peak current. Thus the rms current I_{eff} is equal to $1/\sqrt{2}$ or 0·707 of the *peak* value.

As the electricity is required to do work in some form or another, energy dissipation is the important factor. Thus it is the root mean square (rms) current and voltage which are relevant, and are therefore the quantities which are usually stated. For example, when an alternating supply is stated to be 230 volts this is understood to mean an rms voltage of 230 and therefore a *peak* potential difference (which must be borne by the insulation in the circuit) of 230 $\times$ $\sqrt{2}$ or 325 volts.

The average power dissipation in a resistance can be obtained from the equivalent direct current conditions, being given by the product of the potential difference across the resistance and the current through it. Thus, in the ac case, the average power in watts is given by the product of the rms potential difference in volts and the rms current in amps.*

Circuit Containing Inductance Only

When a *steady* emf is applied to an inductance, it has been explained (p. 172) that an induced emf opposes the rise of the current and operates so long as the current is growing. The *maximum* value attained by the current is determined solely by the applied emf and the resistance of the coil. Consider now the application of an *alternating* emf to a coil having self-inductance but negligible resistance. As a result of the varying current produced by the applied alternating emf, an *induced* emf will be set up which will oppose the current changes. The current variation at any instant must always be such that the induced emf associated with it just balances (i.e. is equal and opposite to) the applied emf. (For, if the applied emf increased more rapidly, there would be a more rapid rise in current which, in turn, would increase the opposing induced emf until a balance was attained.)

Consider now Fig. 90, where the curve *I* shows the variation (against

---

* It should be noted here that in the case of an X-ray tube circuit the effects of cable capacity, non-linearity of tube characteristics, etc., affect the wave form of the current and voltage variations. In this case it is usual to calculate the mean power dissipated in the tube from (rms volts across tube) $\times$ (mean tube current), as this provides the result nearest to measured power values in modern equipments. The *mean* current will in general be recorded by the current meter, and the rms voltage may have to be calculated from the peak voltage as above, assuming a sinusoidal wave form.

time) of the current in the coil. Now, from the discussion in the previous chapter, it appears that the induced emf will be at a maximum when the rate of change of current is at a maximum. Thus, at a time corresponding to a point such as *A*, the current is zero but its *rate of change* is at a maximum, and the induced emf will consequently be at a

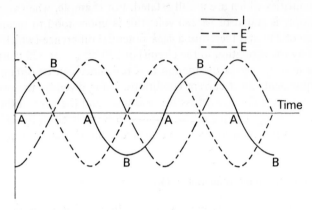

Fig. 90. Alternating emf *E* and current *I* in a circuit containing inductance only. *E'* is the back emf across the inductance.

maximum value (negative or positive according to Lenz's Law, p. 167, to oppose the current change). For a point such as *B*, at the peak of the curve, the current is at a maximum but is momentarily constant, and the induced emf will thus have fallen to zero as there is no changing current in the circuit at this instant. A continuation of this argument yields the curve *E'*, for the variation of the *induced* emf corresponding to the current variation of the curve *I*. Now the *applied* emf will be exactly equal and opposite to *E'*, and will thus be represented by the curve marked *E*. Hence, to sum up, for an alternating emf as shown by curve *E*, the resulting current variation is given by curve *I*, and it is seen that the current follows a curve of an exactly similar *shape* but which is, in time, a quarter of a cycle *behind* the curve of emf.

For a given peak current, the maximum value of the induced emf during the cycle (and hence of the applied emf necessary to produce this current) will depend on the selfinductance *L* of the coil and also on the frequency *f* of the supply (since this will determine the *rate of variation* of the current). Actually, whereas in the resistive circuit the ratio of peak emf to peak current is given by the *resistance* of the circuit, here, in a circuit with inductance only, the ratio is equal to $2\pi fL$ which is known as the *reactance* of the coil, and is usually denoted by X. This is given in *ohms* if the inductance L is in *henries* (p, 172) and the frequency f in *cycles per second*. Thus we have a form of Ohm's Law giving:

$$\text{reactance } X = \frac{\text{peak emf*}}{\text{peak current}}.$$

It must be remembered, however, that in the inductive circuit the peak applied emf and the peak current do not occur at the same instant in time, the current variation lagging in time a quarter of a cycle behind the emf.

The power dissipation at any instant is given by the product of the instantaneous values of applied emf and the current flowing, and will vary as shown in curve W in Fig. 91. It will be seen that this is a cyclic variation with twice the frequency of the current and emf variations.

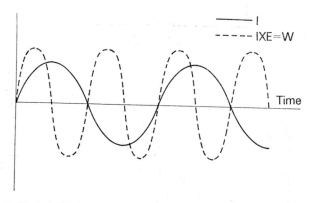

Fig. 91. Variation of power W in a circuit containing inductance only.

It may appear surprising that over part of the cycle the power dissipation is *negative*, but this can be understood in the following physical terms. Because there is no ohmic resistance, there is no conversion of electrical energy to heat within the coil. As the current increases, work is done in establishing the magnetic field associated with this current, corresponding to the *positive* part of the power curve. When the current falls to zero, the magnetic field also falls to zero, and the potential energy stored in the field is recovered and fed back into the circuit, a process which

* Although this result, and those in the following sections, are given in terms of *peak* values (I_0, V_0 and E_0) the relationships do, of course, apply equally to *rms* values (I_{eff}, V_{eff}, and E_{eff}).

corresponds to the *negative* part of the power curve. Thus, as the portions of the curve above and below the axis are exactly equal, the *average* power dissipation over one cycle is zero, and there is no *net* energy consumption from the source in such a circuit containing inductance only.

Circuit Containing Resistance and Inductance in Series

Consider now an alternating emf of peak value E_0 volts applied to a resistance R ohms and an inductance L henries in series (Fig. 92a).

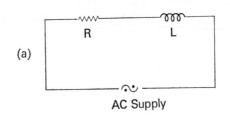

(a)

AC Supply

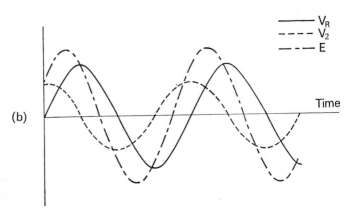

(b)

Fig. 92.

(a) An alternating current circuit containing resistance and inductance in series.

(b) Alternating emf E, and voltages V_R and V_L across resistance and inductance respectively.

An alternating current of peak value I_0 amp will flow in the circuit. The potential difference across the resistance (curve Vz in Fig. 92b) will vary in phase with this current and its peak value V_0 will be given by RI_0. The potential difference across the inductance (curve V_L in Fig. 92b), on the other hand, will be a quarter of a cycle *ahead* of the current variation, and its peak value will be given by $2\pi fLI_0$ (see p. 186). The necessary applied emf will be equal to the sum of these two potential differences (which are not in phase), yielding an emf which varies in the manner shown in curve E, Fig. 92b.

The *peak* (or rms) value of this alternating current is proportional to the *peak* (or rms) value of the applied emf (although they do not occur at the same instant in time). Their *ratio* is again a constant which is referred to in this case as the *impedance* of the circuit.

Thus: $$\frac{\text{peak emf}}{\text{peak current}} = \frac{\text{rms emf}}{\text{rms current}} = \text{constant}$$

$$= \text{impedance of the circuit.}$$

This impedance is said to be in ohms if the emf is in volts and the current in amps. Further it can be shown by calculations (which cannot be included here) that the value of this impedance is given by

$$\sqrt{R^2 + (2\pi fL)^2}, \text{ where } R \text{ is the resistance and}$$
$2\pi fL$ is the reactance of the circuit respectively.

The difference in *phase* between the applied emf and the current obviously depends on the relative values of the resistance and reactance. If the reactance is zero, there is no phase difference, and if the resistance is zero, the current lags one quarter of a cycle behind the applied emf (see p. 186). It is convenient to consider this phase difference as an *angle* expressing the complete cycle difference as $360°$. Then the phase angle (Θ) is given by:

$$\tan \Theta = \frac{\text{reactance}}{\text{resistance}}.$$

Power Factor

It has already been stated (p. 185) that the average power consumption for an alternating current flowing in a circuit containing a resistance only, is given by the product of the rms value of the applied p.d. (V_{eff} volts) and the rms value of the resulting current (I_{eff} amp). Further it has been concluded (p. 188) that there is *no* net consumption of energy (average power is zero) for an alternating current flowing in a 'pure' inductance.

In a circuit containing both resistance and inductance (Fig. 92) the average power will obviously be between these two values, and will depend on the relative values of resistance and reactance. It can be shown that:

Average Power $= (I_{\text{eff}} \cdot V_{\text{eff}}) \times (F)$ watts.

F is known as the *Power Factor* of the circuit and

$$F = \frac{\text{resistance of circuit}}{\text{impedance of circuit}} = \frac{R}{\sqrt{R^2 + (2\pi f L)^2}}$$

Thus, the power factor, F, is *unity* when L is zero, and is *zero* when R is zero, corresponding to the two limiting values of average power given above.

Circuit Containing Capacitor Only

If a capacitor is connected to a source of constant emf, current will flow until the capacitor becomes fully charged (see p. 121). The potential difference V between the plates then equals the applied emf, and the charge stored is given by CV, where C is the capacitance of the capacitor (see p. 114). No further flow of charge can then take place. If, however, the supply is an alternating one, the capacitor will be continually charged and recharged with the opposite polarity. Thus there will be a continual flow of charge into and out of the capacitor, which in fact constitutes an alternating current in the leads to the capacitor, although there is no flow of charge across the dielectric from one plate to the other.

The larger the capacitance of the capacitor the greater the flow of charge during each cycle. Again, the higher the frequency the more rapidly the charging process is completed. Thus the *current* (i.e. rate of flow of charge) for a given alternating emf will increase with both the capacitance C and the frequency f; in fact it can be shown that the *reactance X* of a capacitor is given by $1/2\pi f C$.

Thus, peak emf = (peak current) × (reactance),

or $\qquad E_0 = I_0 \left(\dfrac{1}{2\pi f C} \right).$

The reactance is given in ohms if the capacitance is in farads (p. 114) and the frequency in cycles per second.

The potential difference across the capacitor will follow precisely the applied emf *E*, and the charge *Q* stored in the capacitor will vary in a similar fashion, as shown in Fig. 93. However, the *rate of flow* of charge (i.e. the *current I*) at any time, will be given by the slope of the tangent to curve *Q* at that time. This is obviously at its greatest at points such as *X* and *Y* where the capacitor is discharged and about to be charged again, one way round or the other. When the capacitor is fully charged by the peak applied emf, as at point *Z*, the tangent will be parallel to the time axis and the current, momentarily, will be zero. Thus the current curve will be as shown in curve *I*, Fig. 93, and it is seen that the current variation is a quarter of a cycle *ahead* of the emf.

By an exactly similar argument to that given in the case of an inductance (p. 187), it may be shown that there is no nett power dissipation in a capacitor over a complete cycle, energy being stored in the capacitor during the charging process but recovered during the discharge.

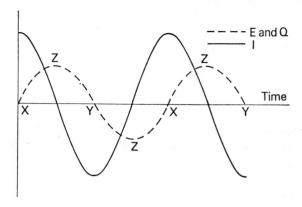

Fig. 93. Alternating emf *E* and current *I* in a circuit containing capacitance only.

Circuit Containing Resistance Inductance and Capacitance in Series

It has been pointed out above that, for a capacitor the variation in the current *leads* the variation in potential difference across the capacitor by one quarter of a cycle. This is the same phase difference (one quarter of a cycle) but in the *opposite sense* to that in a circuit containing a 'pure' inductance (p. 186). In this latter case the current variation *lags* one quarter of a cycle behind that of the potential difference. Therefore the reactance for an inductance and that for a capacitor can be considered to be opposite in *sense*, and these reactances are written with opposite *signs*, as $+ 2\pi fL$ and $- 1/2\pi fC$ respectively. They must be added algebraically (i.e. taking account of sign) to arrive at the *net* reactance of the circuit.

For a circuit containing resistance, inductance and capacitance, the ratio of peak (or rms) applied p.d. to the corresponding peak (or rms) current is, again, a constant (although these two peak values do not, in general, occur at the same instant in time). In this case, the constant ratio is referred to as the *impedance* of the circuit, and is said to be in ohms if the p.d. is in volts and the current in amps. The value of the impedance is given (as on p. 189) by the square root of the sum of the squares of the total resistance and of the total reactance. Here then:

$$\text{Impedance} = \sqrt{R^2 + (2\pi fL - 1/2\pi fC)^2}$$

As before (p. 190), the average power for the circuit is given by:

$$\text{Average power} = V_{\text{eff}} . I_{\text{eff}} . F \text{ watts,}$$

where F is known as the *power factor* for the circuit and is equal to the ratio of the resistance to the impedance (p. 190). Thus we have:

$$F = \frac{R}{\sqrt{R^2 + (2\pi fL - 1/2\pi fC)^2}} .$$

It is apparent that the alternating current flowing in such a circuit can be varied by adjustment of the inductance and capacitance as well as by adjustment of the resistance. In this connection it must be remembered that the higher the inductance the *greater* its reactance (and hence normally the smaller the current for a given emf—but see p. 196) and, in contrast, that the higher the capacitance of any capacitor in the circuit the *lower* its reactance.

Now the inductance of a coil is increased by the use of an iron core. If, then, this core can be moved into and out of the coil, the effective inductance can be varied. This principle is sometimes used to provide a convenient control of current in a circuit at high voltage; for instance, the filament circuit of an X-ray tube. All components of such a circuit are usually at a high voltage with respect to earth, but if a variable inductance of this type is used the current can be safely and easily varied by moving the core (which can be well insulated from the coil) by means of an electric motor. Adjustable inductance cores are also used for 'tuning' (p. 196) in radio and amplifier circuits.

The change of reactance with frequency is also important. A *choke* coil of high inductance will offer only small opposition (owing to its low resistance) to direct current, but its impedance will increase with the frequency of the supply. On the other hand, a capacitor, which will not allow any direct current to pass (having infinitely high reactance at zero frequency), will offer less and less opposition to alternating currents as the frequency rises. These properties are made use of in 'smoothing' circuits (see p. 208, in connection with rectification), where inductances ('chokes') in series, and capacitors in parallel, are used to reduce the alternating 'ripple' of a rectified supply.

Now, although reactances limit the magnitude of the current for a given emf, there is no net power consumption from the source of supply as there would be for a resistance of corresponding value employed for this purpose. This use of reactances to control current without energy loss is sometimes very convenient, but is limited to some extent by the electricity supplier's requirement of the user to keep the power factor (p. 192) of his circuits as a whole as near unity as possible.

An inductance will, of course, always have *some* resistance, and therefore some ohmic loss, and there will also be some hysteresis (p. 87) and eddy current (p. 182) losses in the iron core, but normally these losses will be quite small. A capacitor in which there is a 'leakage' of charge (either through the dielectric or between the terminals) will, in effect, be equivalent to a perfect capacitor with a resistance connected across it, and from the circuit point of view can be treated as such. There will then be some energy loss owing to the leakage current through the 'resistance', and the capacitor will become heated. In general, however, such a condenser would be regarded as faulty and would be replaced.

EXAMPLES

1. A resistance of 100 ohms is connected in series with an inductance of 2 henries and a capacitor of capacitance 7 microfarads across a 230 volt, 50 cycles per sec alternating supply. Calculate the impedance of the circuit, and hence the current, power factor, and energy dissipation in the resistance (π is to be taken as 22/7).

Reactance of inductance $= 2\pi fL$

$$= 2 \times \tfrac{22}{7} \times 50 \times 2$$

$$= 628 \text{ ohms (approx.)}$$

$$\text{Reactance of capacitor} = -\frac{1}{2\pi f C}$$

$$= -\frac{1}{2 \times \frac{22}{7} \times 50 \times 7 \times 10^{-6}}$$

$$= -\frac{10^4}{22}$$

$$= -455 \text{ ohms (approx.)}$$

$$\therefore \text{ total reactance} = +628 - 455$$

$$= +173 \text{ ohms.}$$

$$\therefore \text{ impedance} = \sqrt{(100)^2 + (173)^2}$$

$$= \sqrt{10{,}000 + 30{,}000} \text{ (approx.)}$$

$$= 200 \text{ ohms.}$$

$$\therefore \text{ rms current} = \frac{230}{200}$$

$$= 1 \cdot 15 \text{ amp.}$$

$$\text{Power factor} = \frac{\text{resistance}}{\text{impedance}}$$

$$= \frac{100}{200}$$

$$= 0 \cdot 5$$

$$\therefore \text{ average power dissipation} = (\text{rms volts}) \times (\text{rms amps}) \times (\text{power factor})$$

$$= 230 \times 1 \cdot 15 \times 0 \cdot 5$$

$$= 132 \text{ watts (approx.)}$$

2. A 3 watt lamp designed for operation from a 12 volt supply is to be connected to a 200 volt, 50 cycles per sec alternating supply. Calculate the series capacitance which would be required. Compare the power dissipation in this case with that obtained if a series resistance is used instead of the capacitor.

$$\text{Current (in amps)} \times \text{p.d. (in volts)} = \text{power (in watts)}.$$

$$\therefore \text{ for lamp, current} = \frac{3}{12}$$

$$= \frac{1}{4} \text{ amp.}$$

$$\text{Thus, resistance} = \frac{12}{\frac{1}{4}}$$

$$= 48 \text{ ohms.}$$

Now, emf = current × impedance,

i.e. $200 = \frac{1}{4} \times$ impedance,

∴ required impedance = 4 × 200

$$= 800 \text{ ohms.}$$

Now, (impedance)² = (resistance)² + (reactance)²,

i.e. $640,000 = 2304 + (\text{reactance})^2$,

whence, reactance = $\sqrt{637,696}$

$$= 798 \cdot 5 \text{ ohms.}$$

$$\therefore \frac{1}{2\pi fC} = 798 \cdot 5,$$

$$\text{or } C = \frac{1}{2 \times 798 \cdot 5 \times 3 \cdot 142 \times 50},$$

$$= 4 \times 10^{-6} \text{ farads (approx.)}$$

$$= 4 \text{ microfarads.}$$

Now, in this case, the only power dissipation is that in the lamp, i.e. 3 watts. If a series resistance is used, the total circuit resistance required would be 800 ohms (the value of impedance calculated above), and the power dissipation in this purely resistive circuit would be given by:

$$\text{power} = (\text{rms volts}) \times (\text{rms amps})$$

$$= 200 \times \frac{1}{4}$$

$$= 50 \text{ watts.}$$

EXERCISES

(In all these exercises π may be taken as 22/7.)

1. What is the reactance, at a supply frequency of 50 cycles per sec of a coil of inductance 1·4 henries? What would be the capacitance of a capacitor having the same reactance?

2. When connected to a 120 volt d.c. supply a coil passes a current of 1·33 amp, and when connected to a 240·volts rms, 50 cycles per sec alternating supply the rms current is 1·6 amp.
Calculate the resistance and inductance of the coil, and its power factor for this a.c. supply.

3. The coil of Ex. 2 above is connected in series with a capacitor of capacitance 17 μF. Calculate the circuit impedance and the *peak* current for the 240 volts rms, 50 cycles per sec supply. What is the power factor for this circuit?

Resonance

It will be noticed that a very special case for the value of the impedance of a circuit is obtained when

$$2\pi f L = \frac{1}{2\pi f C}.$$

The *reactance* is then zero. The current is thus limited only by the *resistance* of the circuit which may be (and often is) low, so that extremely high currents (and therefore potential differences across the circuit components) will result. The circuit is said to be *resonant*, and the phenomenon is the electrical analogue of the very large movement of a swing which results when the pushes are timed to fit in exactly with the period of the oscillation, or of the vibration of a musical instrument string when the note to which it is tuned is sounded on another instrument nearby.

The condition for resonance given by the equation above is

$$2\pi f = \frac{1}{\sqrt{LC}}, \text{ or, } f = \frac{1}{2\pi\sqrt{LC}}.$$

For a given frequency the circuit can therefore be made resonant by adjusting L or C (or both) so that $\dfrac{1}{2\pi\sqrt{LC}}$ is numerically equal to the frequency, or, alternatively, for given values of L and C, resonance will occur for the particular frequency of supply given by the expression $\dfrac{1}{2\pi\sqrt{LC}}$. The larger the value of the product LC, the lower the resonant frequency of the circuit.

It is by means of resonance that the very small induced signals from a radio receiving aerial are able to produce currents which can be 'detected' in the circuits 'tuned' to this particular frequency. The radio frequencies are high, so that the values of inductance and capacitance for resonance are quite low. The principle is also used in some X-ray generators in the high voltage (300 to 1000 kV) range. In this case a capacitor is connected across the secondary of the transformer to 'tune' the circuit to the supply frequency (referred to as a *resonant transformer* circuit). Quite a small induced emf in the secondary circuit will then produce a very high current (as the resistance is low), and so a high voltage appears across the capacitor and inductance, and hence across the X-ray tube. The required high voltage on the tube can be obtained with a transformer lacking the usual iron core (being correspondingly lighter) and having a lower mutual inductance. At the usual supply frequency of 50 to 60 cycles per sec the values of inductance and capacity for resonance are inconveniently large, so that for these equipments it is usual to provide a special supply at a higher frequency of say 1000 cycles per sec. (produced by a special alternator driven by an electric motor connected to the normal mains supply).

EXAMPLES

1. A radio circuit consists of a capacitor of capacitance 0·00012 microfarads and an inductance of 40 micro-henries in series with it. To what frequency is the circuit tuned?

$$\text{Resonant frequency} = \frac{1}{2\pi\sqrt{LC}}$$

$$= \frac{1}{2\pi}\sqrt{\frac{1}{120 \times 10^{-12} \times 40 \times 10^{-6}}}$$

$$= \frac{1}{2\pi}\sqrt{\frac{10^{16}}{48}}$$

$$= \frac{10^8}{2\pi \times 6·93}$$

$$= 2·3 \times 10^6 \text{ c/s, or } 2·3 \text{ megacycles per sec.}$$

2. Calculate the inductance which would be necessary in series with a capacitor of capacitance 16 μF to tune the circuit to resonate at a frequency of 50 c/s. Let the inductance required be L henries.

$$\text{Then, resonant frequency} = \frac{1}{2\pi\sqrt{LC}}$$

$$\therefore 50 = \frac{1}{2\pi}\sqrt{\frac{1}{L \times 16 \times 10^{-6}}}$$

$$= \frac{1}{2\pi} \times \frac{10^3}{4}\sqrt{\frac{1}{L}}$$

$$\text{or } L = \left(\frac{10^3}{2\pi \times 4 \times 50}\right)^2$$

$$= 0·63 \text{ henry (approx.).}$$

RECTIFICATION

For many purposes such as heating, lighting and driving motors an alternating current supply is quite satisfactory, but for some uses, such as in X-ray sets or radio and electronic apparatus, it is necessary to have a *direct* current supply, that is, one which at least does not reverse and can, if necessary, be 'smoothed'. Apparatus is therefore required for converting an alternating supply into a direct one. This is carried out by a *rectifier*, the process being known as *rectification*.

Referring back to the discussion of the direct current dynamo (p. 170), it will be noticed that this problem was in fact encountered there, as the direction of the induced emf reversed after half a turn of the coil. In order to avoid the reversal of the voltage supplied by the dynamo, the connections to the coil were reversed at the appropriate point in the rotation by means of a commutator. The commutator is, in fact, a *mechanical rectifier*.

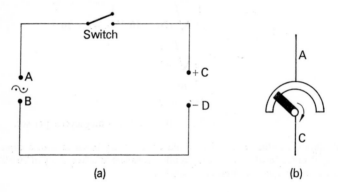

Fig. 94. Principle of the mechanical rectifier.

The basic circuit for a mechanical rectifier is shown in Fig. 94a where an alternating voltage supply is available between *A* and *B*. An external circuit is to be connected to *C* and *D* so that *C* must always be positive (or at least never negative) with respect to *D*. Then, as shown, *B* may be permanently connected to *D*, but *C* is only connected to *A* by operation of the switch during the half cycle when *A* is positive with respect to *B*.

The switch could take the form shown in Fig. 94b in which an arm connected to *C* makes contact with *A* and is rotated by gearing from a synchronous motor to make exactly one revolution in the time of each cycle of voltage. Of course, an actual mechanical switch is not required if a device can be used which will *conduct current in one direction only*. Such a device is referred to as *a rectifier* and is represented diagrammatically in Fig. 95a. In either case, the corresponding variation in voltage across the external circuit *CD* is shown in Fig. 95b.

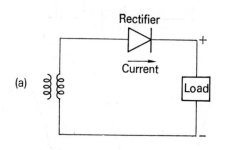

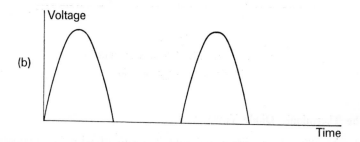

Fig. 95.

(a) Basic circuit for half-wave rectification.

(b) Output voltage variation.

Here only one half of each cycle is utilized, the circuit being effectively disconnected for the other half of the cycle, so this arrangement is said to provide *half-wave rectification*. By suitable connection of other rectifiers, the external circuit can receive voltage with the correct polarity in *both* half cycles of the supply. Such a circuit arrangement (Fig. 96a) provides a voltage variation across the external circuit as shown in Fig. 96b. This is then said to produce *full-wave rectification*. Both these types of rectifier circuit are used to supply voltage to X-ray tubes and examples are described later (p. 205).

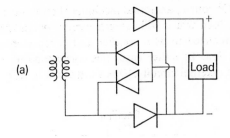

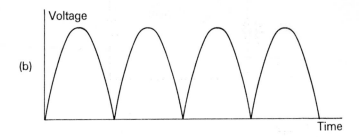

Fig. 96.

(a) Basic circuit for full-wave rectification.

(b) Output voltage variation.

The Thermionic Diode Valve

About 1880 Edison discovered that if a coil of wire (or 'filament'), and a second electrode consisting of a metal plate, were sealed into an evacuated glass bulb, and a current was passed through the filament to bring it to red heat, a flow of charge was possible across the evacuated space from one electrode to the other, provided that the plate (or 'anode') was maintained at a positive potential with respect to the filament (or 'cathode'), but not if this polarity was reversed. That is, the device passed current in one direction only. Because of the similarity in action with a valve in, for instance, a water system, the device became known as an electrical *valve*, in this case a *diode* valve as there were two electrodes. The phenomenon was called the *Edison effect*, and, although no satisfactory explanation was then available, the use of such a device for rectification was immediately obvious. The application of the diode rectifier was particularly due to the work of Fleming.

The effect is now understood in terms of electrons emitted from the surface of a heated electrode, or *thermionic emission* as it is called. In a conductor, although the atoms of the material are fixed in the structure, the outermost ('conduction') electrons are not bound to their atoms, and can in fact easily drift through the material under the influence of a potential difference (however small), thus constituting the flow of electric current. In general there is no net loss of electrons from the conductor when current flows, for, as electrons leave at one end and pass *into* the circuit they are replaced by an equal number of electrons flowing into the conductor at the other end, *from* the circuit. Now it is possible for electrons to escape from the surface of the conductor (in much the same way as some molecules leave the surface of a liquid to form vapour), but for this to happen the electrons must possess a relatively large amount of energy, and at room temperature very few will in fact do so. However, if the conductor is heated the average kinetic energy of the electrons is increased (cf. the kinetic theory of motion of molecules in liquids and gases, p. 2) and a greater number will be able to escape, the emission thus increasing with rising temperature.

The energy which will enable an electron to leave the surface varies with the material, and is known as the 'work function' of that material. Thus, for tungsten, which is commonly used for filament construction in rectifier valves and X-ray tubes, the work function is quite high, being given as 4·55 electron volts (eV). That is, to escape, an electron requires the kinetic energy which it would achieve if accelerated through a potential difference of 4·55 volts. At a temperature of 2000° C the energy of many electrons in the conductor exceeds this, so that a considerable number of electrons will be emitted, and filament temperatures between 2000° and 2500° are usual. The work function of some materials is much lower (the lowest is caesium, 1·75 eV) and it is possible to obtain useful emission at temperatures corresponding to only a dull red heat (700° C) from a surface of barium or strontium oxide, such as is used in some types of radio valve.

Electrons which have already left the surface will repel other electrons which would otherwise have been able to escape, thus reducing the emission; also, some free electrons will be repelled back to the surface. As a consequence a state of equilibrium is reached, with a cloud of electrons, or *space charge* as it is called, surrounding the filament, which is constantly receiving electrons from the filament and returning electrons to it. If, now, a second electrode is placed near to the filament, as in the diode valve, and this second electrode (the *plate* or *anode*) is made positive with respect to the filament, then some of the electrons

14

from the space charge will be attracted to this anode. Thus there will be a flow of negative charge from filament (the *cathode*) to anode, corresponding to the conventional direction of current flow (i.e. a flow of *positive* charge) from anode to cathode.

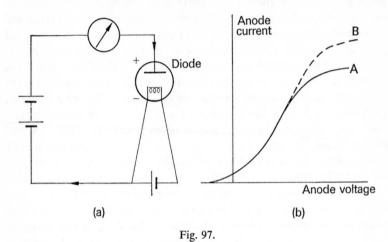

(a)   (b)

Fig. 97.

(a) Circuit for measurement of characteristics of a diode valve.

(b) Characteristic curves for a diode valve.

If the diode valve is connected in the circuit shown in Fig. 97a the variation of this 'anode current' with the potential difference between the electrodes can be illustrated by the *characteristic curve* (as it is called), *A* in Fig. 97b. Even when there is no potential difference, a few of the electrons will in fact still cross to the anode, and there will be a residual anode current. This will be reduced to zero by a small negative potential on the anode, which will cause the electrons to be repelled. As the positive potential (V) on the anode is increased, more and more of the electrons from the space charge are attracted to the anode, and the anode current (I) increases as shown in curve *A*, the relationship being given by:

$$I = V^{3/2} \times \text{constant,}$$

which is often called the *three halves power law*. If the potential difference is increased sufficiently *all* the electrons which are emitted are drawn over to the anode. The current is then no longer 'space charge limited' and cannot increase further; thus the curve flattens out to correspond to this *saturation current*. Increase of the filament temperature (by increasing the heating current through the filament) will increase the emission, but will not affect the current drawn from the space charge for low potential differences. The saturation current will however be higher and will be reached only at a higher potential difference as shown by curve *B*, Fig. 97b.

Now, if a diode valve is to be used as a rectifier the 'resistance' of the valve in the conducting half-cycle should be low. For a point on the first (steep) part of the characteristic (where the current is 'space charge limited'), a large current will be drawn to the anode for a comparatively low anode voltage if the emission is high, so that the effective resistance (voltage across valve/anode current) is low. Under saturation conditions, increase of voltage produces no further increase of current, so that the effective resistance increases. Rectifier valves are therefore operated under 'space charge limited' conditions, so that the normal load current is only a fraction of the saturation current and the effective resistance is low. With the reverse polarity and a good vacuum in the valve the effective resistance is, of course, very high.

It should be noted that, although an X-ray tube is essentially a form of diode valve (with a heated filament emitting electrons which are attracted to an anode), the requirements are different. The purpose here is to accelerate electrons through a *large* potential difference. Thus the tube is required to carry a limited current (to avoid over-heating of the anode) with a very large potential difference between the electrodes (i.e. a *high* effective resistance). Further, the tube current should be variable for a given voltage across the tube by alteration of the filament heating current. The X-ray tube is, therefore, usually operated under conditions approximating to saturation, although this may not apply fully over the whole range of working voltage or in some very high current (radiographic) tubes.

Conversely, as there is no essential difference between a diode valve and an X-ray tube, X-rays will be produced in the diode valve by the electron bombardment of the anode. As has been pointed out, the voltage across a diode valve is designed to be low, so that the X-ray output will normally be low and of very 'soft' (i.e. easily absorbed) radiation. A form of construction which has sometimes been adopted makes use of a cylindrical metal anode surrounding the filament, the latter lying along the axis of the cylinder. This provides a large anode surface area for heat dissipation and also ensures that most of the X-rays are absorbed in passing through the anode. Thus, in practice, the X-ray emission from rectifier valves does not represent a hazard.

Solid-State Rectifiers

Apart from the thermionic diode valve, a number of solid conductor devices are available which will act as rectifiers, that is, they will only allow current to flow in one direction, or at least the resistance is very much lower for conduction in one direction than the other.

The earliest form consisted of a layer of *copper oxide* formed on a copper sheet. Then the conventional flow of current (from positive to negative) takes place with low resistance from the outer oxide surface through to the copper (i.e. at right angles to the plane of the sheet). But a high resistance is offered to flow in the reverse direction. With this device, only a small potential difference can be maintained across an individual rectifier and, for efficient operation, any temperature rise must be limited. Thus it is usual for a number of such rectifier elements to be mounted in series, with spacers and cooling fins in between. With large plate areas, the copper oxide rectifier is then particularly useful for rectification of high currents at fairly low voltages.

More recently *selenium* rectifiers, which provide rectification at the interface between layers of selenium and iron or aluminium, and *silicon* crystal rectifiers have been developed. As these can operate with higher voltages across each unit and at higher temperature, it is possible to use such rectifiers in place of valves in X-ray generator circuits. Solid-state rectifiers, of course, require no filament heating supply and have a long useful life. Thus they are likely to be used to an increasing extent in new X-ray generating equipment.

RECTIFIER CIRCUITS

The Self-Rectified Circuit—Half-Wave Rectification

The fact that the X-ray tube is equivalent to a diode valve, in that it will pass current in one direction only, means that it can act as its own rectifier. In the so-called *self-rectified* circuit, the X-ray tube is connected straight across the secondary coil of the transformer, as shown in Fig. 98. When A is positive with respect to B, current will flow through the tube, but in the other half-cycle no current will flow, that is, the tube provides half-wave rectification. A disadvantage of this simple circuit is that during the non-conducting half-cycle, the secondary voltage which appears across the tube (the *inverse* voltage) is higher than that obtained during the conducting half-cycle, when the load current leads to losses in the transformer and a secondary voltage lower than on 'open circuit' (see transformer regulation, p. 179). Thus the insulation of the tube, tube support and cables must all stand this inverse voltage, which is higher than the voltage at which the tube is actually producing

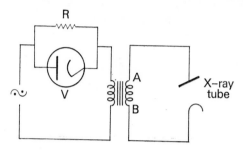

R

Fig. 98. The self-rectified X-ray generator circuit.

X-rays. To reduce this inverse voltage some manufacturers use a high-current rectifier valve (V in Fig. 98) in the primary circuit of the transformer. During the half-cycle in which the tube is conducting this valve also conducts, and offers only a low resistance in the primary circuit. In the reverse half-cycle, this rectifier does not conduct, and the primary current must pass through the resistance R connected in parallel with the rectifier valve. This leads to a reduction in the voltage across the primary of the transformer, and thus to a lower secondary voltage during this half-cycle. That is, the inverse voltage on the tube is reduced, so that it is not at any rate *greater* than the tube voltage in the conducting half-cycle.

This circuit is simple and cheap, and is quite commonly used. It does not require any high-voltage rectifier valves, and if the transformer and X-ray tube are mounted together in an oil-filled tank, the high-voltage part of the circuit is compact and no (expensive) high-voltage cables are required. It does, however, only offer half-wave rectification (see Fig. 95b).

Full-Wave Rectification

To provide full-wave rectification of the voltage applied to an X-ray tube, it is usual to connect four valves in the so-called *bridge* circuit shown in Fig. 99 (cf. Fig. 96a). During the half-cycle when the end X

of the transformer secondary coil is positive, and the end *Y* negative, current will pass through the rectifier *A*, the X-ray tube and the rectifier *D*, rectifiers *B* and *C* not conducting. During the next half-cycle current

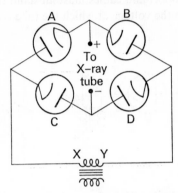

Fig. 99. The four valve bridge circuit.

will reach the X-ray tube via rectifiers *B* and *C*. Thus the voltage applied to the tube will follow the full-wave rectified form shown in Fig. 96b (p. 200)* and the tube will be operating during both half-cycles.

This bridge circuit, with two pairs of rectifiers being used in alternate half-cycles, is particularly useful where high X-ray tube currents are required (with consequent over-heating of the rectifier anodes as a problem), for instance in a radiographic unit.

Constant-Potential Rectifier Circuits

Either metal rectifiers or thermionic valves may be used in the half-wave and full-wave rectifier circuits shown in Fig. 95a (p. 199) and Fig. 96a (p. 200). However, the output of these circuits, although uni-directional, is not constant, and in order to provide a fairly constant voltage supply a *smoothing* circuit must be used. Thus a capacitor connected across the 'load' (Fig. 100a), is charged up by the current flowing through the rectifier in the conducting half-cycle. As the applied voltage falls, and

---

* For full-wave rectification of a sine wave of peak value V_0 the *mean rectified* voltage can be shown to be equal to $2V_0/\pi$. For *half*-wave rectification the average, or mean rectified, value over one cycle of the sine wave will obviously be half this or V_0/π, as alternate half-cycles are missing. These mean rectified values should not be confused with the rms values discussed on p. 184.

during the next half-cycle, the capacitor discharges through the load, thus maintaining the current through the latter. As the capacitor discharges, the voltage across it (and across the load) falls, and therefore the load current falls. However, if the capacitance of the capacitor is large, the charge lost during the half-cycle will lead to a small drop only in the capacitor voltage before it is recharged (Fig. 100b), so that the *ripple* on the voltage applied to the load is only a fraction of the peak value.

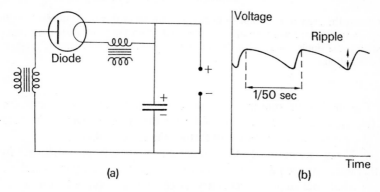

Fig. 100a and b. The constant voltage rectifier circuit.

An analogy here may prove useful. We may imagine a water storage tank (the 'capacitor') being *supplied* with water from a pump, in a series of regularly spaced 'gushes' (the half-cycles during which the rectifier is conducting). The water is being *taken* from the tank all the time, and the 'head' of water (i.e. the depth of the water in the tank) determines the supply pressure ('voltage'). This will be *'topped up'* by each gush, but will *fall* between gushes, this rise and fall in the water level in the tank representing the 'ripple' in the supply pressure. Clearly the magnitude of this variation (or 'ripple') will depend on the volume of the tank (the 'capacity' of the capacitor) and the rate at which water is being drained away (i.e. the load 'current').

EXAMPLE

In an X-ray generator providing half-wave rectification, a capacitor, capacitance 0·02 μF, connected across the tube, is charged to a peak voltage of 100 kV. If the current taken by the X-ray tube is 10 mA, what is the approximate value of the voltage ripple?

For a supply at 50 cycles per sec the capacitor is recharged to the peak voltage every fiftieth of a second, so, approximately, we have to calculate the drop in the voltage across the capacitor as a result of providing a current of 10 mA for 1/50 sec.

$$\text{Now, voltage} = \frac{\text{charge in coulombs}}{\text{capacity in farads}} \qquad \text{(see p. 114)}$$

$$= \frac{10 \times 10^{-3} \times 0\cdot02}{0\cdot02 \times 10^{-6}}$$

= 10,000 volts, or 10 % of the peak value.

Actually the capacitor will not be discharging for all of this time interval of 1/50 sec, as its recharge will take up a short period. Thus the result above will over-estimate the ripple voltage, but the calculation provides an approximate value of the variation.

This method of smoothing can of course also be adapted for use with a full-wave rectifier circuit, in which case the more frequent recharging of the capacitor will reduce still further the ripple voltage.

In X-ray circuits no further smoothing is usually provided, but in other apparatus requiring a very constant voltage (e.g. amplifiers, radios, etc.) additional steps are necessary. A *choke* coil is connected in series with the load across the smoothing capacitor (Fig. 101). As the load

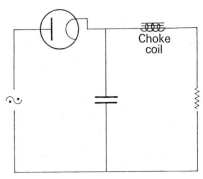

Fig. 101. Constant-potential rectifier circuit with 'choke' coil smoothing.

current varies, the induced emf set up in this inductance acts to oppose the changes and so help to smooth the supply. An alternative description of the action of the smoothing circuit can be given by considering the total current as made up of an alternating component super-imposed on a constant current. The inductance then increases the impedance of the load circuit to this alternating current, which finds a low impedance path through the large capacitance capacitor connected in parallel. In, for instance, an amplifier the capacitance of the smoothing capacitor will be 8 to 32 μF, and the choke coil will have an inductance of 2 to 10 henries. In X-ray circuits, because of the high voltage used, the capacitors become very bulky, and capacitances of 0·01 or 0·02 μF only are practicable.

A second smoothing capacitor may also be connected directly across the load. This will act as a reservoir of charge, still further reducing the variations in the final load current.

Voltage Doubling Circuits

Doubling the step-up ratio necessitates a very considerable increase in the weight and size of a transformer, and so, in the production of a very high voltage, it is convenient to make use of circuits which provide output voltages twice that of the transformer secondary coil. A number of these circuits have been used in X-ray generators but only the so-called *Greinacher circuit* (Fig. 102) will be described in detail. This

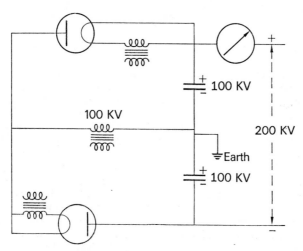

Fig. 102. The Greinacher circuit.

provides voltage-doubling and also a constant-voltage output, and is still used in most constant-voltage generators. There are two capacitors connected in series across the tube with their centre point earthed. The transformer is then connected so as to provide a half-wave rectifier circuit charging up each capacitor in turn (through the appropriate rectifier valve), during alternate half-cycles. Thus each capacitor charges up to the peak voltage of the transformer, say 100 kV, and the sum of these two capacitor voltages will then have a peak value of about 200 kV, with a small ripple, usually of about 10 per cent of this peak value.

A meter to read the current flowing through the X-ray tube is often connected as shown in Fig. 102. In this position the meter itself is at the high voltage of the anode of the tube, and so cannot be safely mounted on the operator's control panel. In the older equipments making use of this circuit the meter was viewed at a distance through a window in the generator room—an inconvenient arrangement. It is possible by using a bridge rectifier circuit in association with the meter itself, to incorporate the latter in the Greinacher circuit between one end of the secondary winding of the transformer and the earthed centre point of the condensers, thus enabling the meter to be mounted on the control panel. More modern sets use a double Greinacher circuit, which also enables the meter to be at earth potential.

THE TRIODE VALVE

Although this section is not concerned with rectification, it conveniently follows a discussion of the thermionic diode valve.

It was pointed out in that discussion that, under normal conditions of operation, there remains a 'space charge' of electrons near the cathode. De Forest in 1907 was the first valve engineer to make use of a third electrode (thus making it a *triode* valve), consisting of a grid of fine wires placed between the cathode and anode in this region of space charge. It is found that very small changes in the potential of such a *grid* electrode causes very marked changes in the number of electrons reaching the anode (i.e. in the anode current). If then the anode current is passed through a resistance, this current change will produce a change in the voltage of the anode, and we find that a *small* change of voltage on the grid can produce a *large* voltage change on the anode, that is, the valve functions as an amplifier of voltage changes. The triode valve therefore proves to be very valuable in electrical measuring equipment, amplifiers and radios, and in electronic apparatus generally. Valves with several such grids (*tetrode, pentode,* etc., valves) are also used now, but we shall restrict the discussion here to the triode valve.

As with the diode valve, we may represent the operation of the triode valve by its characteristic curves. These can take two forms. It is usual to operate the valve at some definite filament voltage and not to consider changes in this supply. However, we may still consider changes in anode current with grid voltage at a series of constant anode voltages (*grid* or *mutual* characteristics) as shown in Fig. 103a, or alternatively they may be drawn to show the variation of anode current with anode voltage at a series of constant grid voltages (*anode* characteristics) as shown in Fig. 103b. Such measurements can be made with an arrangement of batteries and meters as shown in Fig. 103c. It will be seen from Fig. 103a that, over a considerable range, the relationship between anode current and grid voltage is a linear one, and the curves for various anode voltages are nearly parallel. The slope of these lines (i.e. the anode current change, in milliamps, per volt change in grid potential) is known as the *mutual conductance* (g_m) of the valve. For different types of triode valve this mutual conductance will vary from about 1 to 8 mA/V.

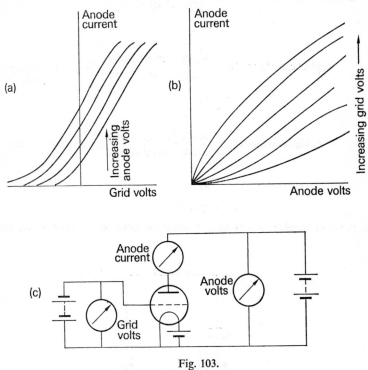

Fig. 103.

(a) Mutual characteristic curves for a triode valve.

(b) Anode characteristic curves for a triode valve.

(c) Circuit for measurement of characteristics of triode valve.

From the series of curves it is possible to read off the change in anode potential (in volts) which at constant grid potential will produce some specified anode current change (say 1 mA), and also the change in grid voltage at constant anode potential to produce the same anode current change. The ratio of these two voltage changes is known as the *amplification factor* (μ) of the valve, and may vary from about 5 to 100.

A third valve 'constant' R_a is known as the *anode resistance* (or sometimes *slope* resistance) which is the ratio of the change in anode voltage to the corresponding change in anode current (in amps) for a constant grid voltage. This ratio can be expressed in the same units as resistance, that is, ohms, and may range from 1000 to 50,000 ohms.

These three valve constants are, of course, closely related.

$$\text{Thus, mutual conductance } (g_m) = \frac{\text{anode current change}}{\text{grid voltage change}}, \text{anode voltage constant}$$

$$= \frac{i_a}{v_g},$$

$$\text{amplification factor } (\mu) = \frac{\text{anode voltage change}}{\text{grid voltage change}}, \text{ for the same change in anode current}$$

$$= \frac{v_a}{v_g},$$

$$\text{anode resistance } (R_a) = \frac{\text{anode voltage change}}{\text{anode current change}}, \text{grid voltage constant}$$

$$= \frac{v_a}{i_a}.$$

$$\therefore \; \mu = g_m \cdot R_a,$$

or, in words, amplification factor = (mutual conductance) × (anode resistance).

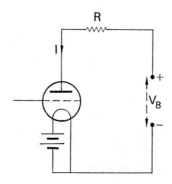

Fig. 104. Basic circuit of triode valve used as a voltage amplifier.

If now we consider a simple circuit, as in Fig. 104, with a resistance R ohms connected to the anode of the valve, then, if the anode current is I amps, and the anode (high tension) battery voltage is V_B, the actual voltage of the anode will be $(V_B - I \cdot R)$.

A small increase of v_g volts in the potential of the grid (i.e. one over which gm is constant) will produce a *rise* in anode current, and consequently a *fall* in anode voltage. That is, in such a circuit a change in grid potential affects both anode current and anode voltage. For small changes it is possible to consider the effect of grid and anode voltage changes separately, and add the corresponding current changes. Thus, if i_A is the resultant change in anode current,

$$i_A = \text{(change due to grid voltage change } v_g,$$
$$\text{with constant anode voltage)}$$
$$+ \text{ (change due to anode voltage change } v_A,$$
$$\text{with constant grid voltage)}$$
$$= v_g \cdot gm + v_A/R_a.$$

Now the change in anode voltage is due to the change in anode current flowing through the resistance R, an *increase* in current leading to a *fall* in anode voltage.

$$\therefore v_A = -i_A R,$$

$$\text{or } i_A = -\frac{v_A}{R}.$$

Substituting this value of i_A in the equation above gives

$$-\frac{v_A}{R} = v_g gm + \frac{v_A}{R_a}.$$

Whence, $\quad -v_A\left(\frac{1}{R} + \frac{1}{R_a}\right) = v_g gm$.

Thus, voltage amplification of the circuit

$$\frac{v_A}{v_g} = \frac{-gm}{\left(\dfrac{1}{R} \quad \dfrac{1}{R_a}\right)}$$

$$= \frac{-gm}{\dfrac{1}{R_a}\left(1 + \dfrac{R_a}{R}\right)}$$

$$= -\frac{gm R_a}{\left(1 + \dfrac{R_a}{R}\right)}$$

Substituting for $gm R_a$, $\quad \dfrac{v_A}{v_g} = -\dfrac{\mu}{\left(1 + \dfrac{R_a}{R}\right)}$.

This will always be numerically less than μ, the amplification factor of the valve, but will approach this value if R, the circuit resistance, is large compared with R_a, the anode resistance of the valve.

It should be stressed again that a *rise* in grid potential leads to a *fall* in anode potential, so that although there is an increase in *amplitude* of the voltage variation in passing through the valve, there is also a change in *sign* or *phase*. This is the meaning of the minus sign in the expression derived above for the voltage amplification of the circuit.

CHAPTER 12

Waves and the Propagation of Radiant Energy

CYCLIC CHANGE AND WAVE PROPAGATION

We are all familiar with the circular ripples (or 'waves') which spread outwards across the smooth surface of a pond from the point at which a stone has entered. These waves give the impression that there is a bodily movement of water away from the point of the disturbance. That this is not so is easily demonstrated by the behaviour of a cork or similar light object floating on the water in the path of the waves. If there were a bodily flow of water the cork would be carried along, but this does not happen; instead, the cork bobs up and down (there is also a slight to-and-fro movement), its position on the pond remaining unaltered after the waves have passed.

The fact that a wave does not carry matter along with it is perhaps even more strikingly demonstrated by the 'waves' which may be made to pass along a rope lying stretched out on the ground. If one end is shaken quickly up and then down again, the hump or 'crest' of a wave is seen to move along the length of the rope, but obviously the *material* of the rope itself does not travel with the wave. It is a *disturbance* which travels along, resulting from the fact that a succession of points along the rope, one after the other, go through a complete cycle of movement, each point rising then falling again.

This transmission of a cyclic change is characteristic of *wave* propagation, and is perhaps most clearly illustrated by means of a model (Fig. 105). A handle *H* rotates a shaft (not seen in Fig. 105) which has a series of cranks in it rather like the crankshaft of an engine comprised of many cylinders. Each crank is attached by means of a 'connecting rod' to a series of 'pistons' *A*, *B*, *C*, *D*, etc. The holes in the guides through which *A*, *B*, *C*, *D*, etc., pass constrain the 'pistons' to move up and down in vertical lines only, as the crankshaft is rotated. Each 'piston' carries a knob on it to make its up-and-down movements more conspicuous. As *H* is turned, each knob performs the same cycle of up-and-down movements, but as the cranks operating *A*, *B*, *C*, *D*, etc., are arranged to have constant angular differences in their orientations round the axis of the shaft (forming, in effect, a spiral of cranks as one passes along the shaft), it follows that as, for example, knob *I* rises and falls, knob *J* (performing the same cycle of motion) lags slightly behind knob *I* as it does so. Similarly, knob *K* lags behind *J*, *L* behind *K*, and so on. Two important points are to be noted:

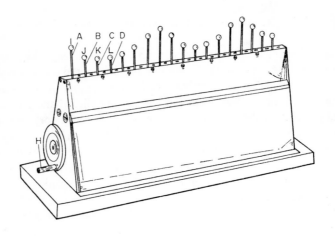

Fig. 105. A model illustrating the principle of propagation of a transverse wave motion.

(1) At any instant in their motions the knobs have the general appearance shown in Fig. 105; they depict, as it were, a series of *wave* crests and troughs.

(2) As the knobs rise and fall in the manner described, this series of crests and troughs moves steadily along (e.g. from left to right), in spite of the fact that the knobs themselves move only up and down. Reversing the direction of rotation of *H*, thereby causing *I* to lag behind *J*, *J* behind *K*, and so on, reverses the *direction* in which the 'waves' appear to travel.

Thus we may conclude that the propagation of a train of waves is associated with the occurrence of a regular cycle (e.g. of motion) at a series of points along the line of propagation, the cyclic changes at the series of points being related to each other in such a way that the stage in the cycle (known as the 'phase', see also Chap. 11) obtaining at any point, differs by a constant amount from that obtaining at the neighbouring points to the left or right (the points being imagined to be spaced out at regular intervals along the line which constitutes the direction of propagation of the wave motion). If the cyclic changes associated with the waves take place in a direction at right angles to the direction of propagation of the waves (as in the case of the ripples on the pond, the waves along a rope, or the 'waves' associated with the motion of the knobs described above) the waves are said to be *transverse*.

If, on the other hand, the cyclic changes take place in the *same* direction as that of the wave, the waves are called '*longitudinal*'. For example, if a long spiral spring composed of light wire be supported at a number of points along its length by cotton threads, one end of the spring can be pushed and pulled suddenly, causing the spring to be first compressed and then extended. Regions of compression, each followed by a region of 'extension', are seen to travel along the spring, and if the latter is watched closely it is seen that the mechanism by which these 'waves' are transmitted consists of the successive to-and-fro movements of individual turns of the spring *along the line of travel of the waves*, i.e. the latter comprise a *longitudinal* wave motion. The transmission of sound provides an important example of a longitudinal wave motion, consisting of alternating regions of compression and rarefaction transmitted through the air by the gas molecules taking up a to-and-fro motion in the direction in which the sound is travelling.

ELECTROMAGNETIC WAVES

In this group are a number of very important forms of radiation, including radio, heat, light and also the X- and gamma-rays used in radiology.

To understand their nature let us consider again the model shown in Fig. 105. We might suppose that at any instant the displacement of a particular knob from the point representing its mean position denoted, in both magnitude and direction, the instantaneous strength of the *electric field* obtaining at that point. Suppose that at a certain moment the knobs occupied the positions L, M, . . ., T etc. (Fig. 106a), their mean positions being A, B, . . ., I. Then AL would represent in magnitude and direction the electric field value at point A at the particular instant considered, *BM* the electric field at *B*, *CN* the field at *C*, and so on. In passing, it is to be noted that, momentarily, at *E*, there is *no* electric field, whilst at *F*, *G*, etc., the fields are opposite in direction to those at *A*, *B*, *C*, etc.

After an exceedingly short time interval, we may suppose that the electric field value at *A* has fallen to zero, whilst that at *E* has grown from zero to the value represented by *EP*, the fields at the other points having changed in the manner indicated (Fig. 106b). In practice one must envisage an infinite number of points along the line *ABCD*, at all

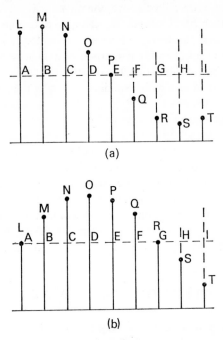

Fig. 106.

of which there are electric fields fitting in with the values shown at *A*, *B*, *C*, *D*, etc. If, then, we imagine all these fields undergoing the cyclic changes in both magnitude and direction indicated by the motion of the knobs of the model of Fig. 105, we shall have a 'transverse' electric wave travelling along the line on which *A*, *B*, *C*, *D* etc. lie.

In an *electromagnetic* wave there is also a transverse *magnetic* wave, coupled, so to speak, with the electric wave, the plane containing the oscillating magnetic fields being at right angles to that containing the electric fields. Thus in Fig. 107 (which gives a 'perspective' view), the vertical plane indicated contains, say, the electric field directions, whilst the horizontal plane contains the magnetic field directions, the direction of propagation of the electromagnetic wave being along the line *XY* common to both planes. Thus, at some particular instant, the electric field at point *A* on *XY* is indicated by *AM* (vertically upwards) whilst the associated magnetic field at this point is denoted by *AN* (a horizontal line which must be imagined to be coming *out* of the paper). At the same instant, at some point *B* further along *XY*, the electric field *BO* is vertically downwards, whilst the magnetic field *BP* is horizontal and directed *into* the paper. Further along still (at *C*) the directions associated with point *A* apply once more. If we then imagine two sets of knobs, one set lying along the full curve (i.e. the vertical plane), and representing *electric* field values, and the other set lying along the dotted curve (i.e.

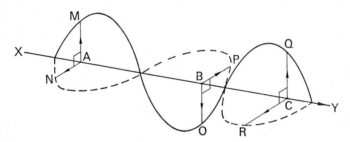

Fig. 107. 'Perspective view' of electric and magnetic field variations in an electromagnetic radiation wave motion.

the horizontal plane) representing *magnetic* field values, the knobs performing in their respective planes the same motions as before, we can form some mental picture of the manner in which the associated transverse electric and magnetic fields vary during the propagation of an *electromagnetic* wave.

WAVELENGTH, FREQUENCY AND VELOCITY

There are certain aspects of wave propagation which must be discussed briefly at this point.

Wavelength

Since 'transverse' waves are the only ones which we shall study here, we may define 'wavelength' as the length occupied by one complete 'crest' and 'trough' (Fig. 108).

It is useful to appreciate that 'wavelength' may also be defined as the distance between any two consecutive points along the wavetrain *at which the cyclic changes* (e.g. of electric and magnetic fields) *always remain in step* (or as is usually said, are always *in phase*). Thus, in Fig. 108, the values at *A*, *B* and *C* are momentarily zero, whilst a short time afterwards, corresponding to the dotted line, they have the values indicated by *AP*, *BQ*, and *CR*, and are therefore equal to each other and all directed downwards. By drawing still further diagrams with the wavetrain displaced more and more to the right it can easily be shown that the conditions at *A*, *B* and *C* continue to be in step with each other, thus satisfying the definition that the distances between *A* and *B*, and *B* and *C*, are each equal to one wavelength. It is then easy to see why points *W* and *Y* (Fig. 108) do not fit in with *A*, *B* and *C*, for, in the dotted curve the displacements *WX* at *W* and *YZ* at *Y*, though *equal* to those at *A*, *B* and *C*, are directed *upwards*.

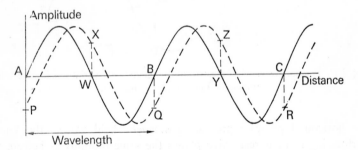

Fig. 108.

From all this it follows that *the passage of one complete wave past any point on the line of propagation results in one complete cycle of changes at that point* (for example, by the time that part of the wave which is at *A* has reached *B*, the changes at *B* begin repeating themselves, and so on).

It is conventional to denote wavelength by the Greek letter λ (pronounced lambda), and it will obviously be measured in units of length. Thus, for radio waves the wavelength is stated in metres or centimetres, but for light, X-rays, etc., the use of the centimetre leads to inconveniently small numbers. Therefore a number of other smaller units have been defined, and the wavelength is usually given in the unit which proves to be the most convenient. These are:

the micron (written μ) $= 1/1000$ mm (or 10^{-4} cm),*
the angstrom* unit (written Å) $= 10^{-8}$ cm,*
and the X unit $= 10^{-11}$ cm.
Thus 1 Å $= 1000$ X units,
$1 \mu = 10,000$ Å,
and 1 cm $= 10,000 \mu$.

Frequency

For any given wavetrain the frequency may be defined as the number of complete waves which pass any fixed point in the path of the waves in unit time. It is obviously also equal to the number of complete waves *emitted* by the source in unit time.

Frequency is usually denoted by the Greek letter ν (pronounced *nu*) or the English letter n, and is measured in *cycles per second* (or Hertz, Hz).

Velocity

This may be defined as the distance traversed by the waves in unit time, and is usually denoted by V.

Thus, under ordinary atmospheric conditions, sound emitted by one person would, in one second, just reach another person 1080 feet away, and the velocity of sound is therefore said to be 1080 feet per second (329 m per sec).

As sound is transmitted by means of the movement of the particles of the medium, a material medium is necessary, and transmission is not possible *in vacuo*. However, in the case of electromagnetic waves this is not so, and, in fact, as has been pointed out before, the heat and light from the sun travel through free space for almost their entire journey to the Earth. All electromagnetic radiations, whatever their nature, travel through free space with a velocity of 186,000 miles per second (3×10^{10} cm per sec.). This particular velocity is usually denoted by the letter c.

Thus, $c = 3 \times 10^{10}$ cm per sec (3×10^{8} m per sec).

* The micron also corresponds to one micro-metre (μm $= 10^{-6}$m) and 10Å corresponds to one nano-metre (nm $= 10^{-9}$m). These are units recommended in the S. I. system.

The Relationship between λ, ν and V

Suppose a wavetrain, the source of which is at O, has attained a length OP after travelling for unit time. Then the *number* of waves between O and P is equal to the *frequency* ν. The total length of the wavetrain between O and P is ν × λ, and since this is the distance travelled by the radiation in unit time, it is numerically equal to the velocity V.

Hence, $V = \nu\lambda$.

THE ELECTROMAGNETIC SPECTRUM

It is usual to refer to the 'colours of the spectrum', by which are meant the components of 'white' light. They are generally named (in order) as violet, indigo, blue, green, yellow, orange and red. In actual fact these constitute a small group of electromagnetic radiations covering almost exactly a two-to-one range of wavelengths (or frequencies). At one end of the range is violet with the shortest wavelength of approximately 4000 Å (and thus the highest frequency), and at the other end is red, with a wavelength just short of 8000 Å (with a frequency approximately half that of violet radiation). The difference between colours of the visible spectrum are due to their different frequencies (or wavelengths).

Now the different notes on a musical instrument, a piano for example, are also associated with differences of frequency (or wavelength—once they have become sound waves travelling through the surrounding air), and two notes an octave apart have a frequency of 2 : 1. For example, if middle C has a frequency of 256 cycles per sec, the C an octave above has a frequency of 512 cycles per sec, and the C an octave below a frequency of 128 cycles per sec, and so on. The very wide range of musical sounds employed by a composer (from the deepest bass notes of an organ to the shrillest notes of the piccolo) are accommodated within a range of eight octaves or so. In comparison, Table VI presents a chart of the whole spectrum of electromagnetic radiations, and it is seen that visible light occupies one 'octave' among some sixty 'octaves' over which the whole spectrum extends. It will also be seen that the X-, and gamma, radiations used in radiology represent about one sixth of the total number of octaves in the spectrum.

In the left-hand column the radiations are listed in order of decreasing wavelength (or increasing frequency) beginning with radio waves, the longest of which have wavelengths of the order of thousands of metres, decreasing, as already noted, to a few centimetres in the case of 'radar' (or a few millimetres under laboratory conditions), and continuing with infra-red, visible, ultra-violet, X-, gamma and some cosmic radiations. The other columns indicate approximate frequency and wavelength

TABLE VI

The Electromagnetic Spectrum

Radiation Type	Wavelength	Frequency (cycles per sec.)
Long & medium wave radio	30000 — 100 metres	$10^4 — 3 \times 10^6$
Short wave radio	100 — 1 metre	$3 \times 10^6 — 3 \times 10^8$
Radar & microwave radio	1 metre — 1 mm or less	$3 \times 10^8 — 3 \times 10^{11}$
Infra-red (heat) radiation	100 microns — 8000 Å	$3 \times 10^{12} — 3 \cdot 75 \times 10^{14}$
Visible light	8000 — 4000 Å	$3 \cdot 75 \times 10^{14} — 7 \cdot 5 \times 10^{14}$
Ultra-violet radiation	4000 — 1000 Å	$7 \cdot 5 \times 10^{14} — 3 \times 10^{15}$
Grenz rays (very long wavelength X-rays)	10 — 0·5 Å	$3 \times 10^{17} — 6 \times 10^{18}$
Superficial (& diagnostic) X-rays	0·5 — 0·1 Å	$6 \times 10^{18} — 3 \times 10^{19}$
Deep therapy X-rays	0·1 — 0·03 Å (100 — 30 X units)	$3 \times 10^{19} — 10^{20}$
Gamma rays	0·1 — 0·006 Å (100 — 6 X units)	$3 \times 10^{19} — 5 \times 10^{20}$
Megavoltage X-rays	0·03 — 0·0001 Å (30 — 0·1 X units)	$10^{20} — 3 \times 10^{22}$
Some Cosmic rays	Down to about 0·2 X unit	Up to about 15×10^{22}

ranges, the latter being given in units appropriate to the particular radiation.

Radiation Energy: Photons

All the radiations listed in Table VI are electromagnetic in nature and differ only in their frequencies (and corresponding wavelengths). However, their mechanisms of interaction and the effects which they produce are very different indeed. This can be understood in terms of the so-called *Quantum Theory of Radiation* first proposed by Einstein. For any given radiation, energy can only be emitted or interact with matter in certain *units*, referred to as *quanta* or *photons* of this radiation. The *amount* of energy in this basic unit is proportional to the *frequency* of the radiation (and so is inversely proportional to its wavelength).

Thus, although the same total energy may be carried by either a radio or an X-ray beam, as the frequency of X-radiation is some 10^{12} times greater, the *photon energy* will be correspondingly higher. Hence, this very much greater amount of energy will be involved in each X-ray interaction and much more significant effects will be observed from the events. For instance, electrons may be detached from atoms (the atoms are *ionized*), molecular bonds may be broken and important biochemical changes may result.

Also, if an energy change in an atom results in the emission of radiation, this energy will constitute a *single photon* (unit of energy) with a corresponding frequency for the radiation. Again a high photon energy would correspond to X-radiation and a lower photon energy to visible light or heat emission. These concepts are found to be very significant in the study of radiology.

RECTILINEAR PROPAGATION

If we have what may be termed, for all practical purposes, a *point source* (e.g. an electric lamp with a very small filament, or an X-ray tube in which the X-rays emanate from an area of metal only one sq mm or so in area) then the radiation from it may be considered to consist of *spherical* electromagnetic disturbances, spreading out in all directions from the source with a velocity of 3×10^{10} cm per sec. That is to say, the *radius* of such a spherical disturbance will, after one second, be 300,000,000 metres, and after 2 seconds, 600,000,000 metres and so on. This spreading out of *spherical* waves from a point source may be compared with the *circular* waves on water discussed at the beginning of this chapter, but in the present case the phenomenon is a three dimensional one, whilst the water waves are propagated in two dimensions only.

If, now, we imagine ourselves able to observe a single point such as *A* (Fig. 109) on a spherical wave as the latter spreads outwards from the source at *O*, then it would successively pass through such points as *B, C, D*, etc., on the straight line *OP*. Now *OP* is referred to as a *ray*, and may be defined as the path taken by a small element of a *wave*, as the latter travels through space. The fact that *rays* (such as *OP*) are *straight* is the origin of the expression 'light travels in straight lines'.*

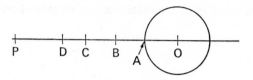

Fig. 109. A spherical wave motion spreading out from *O*. *OP* represents a 'ray'.

So also do X-rays and gamma-rays, and therefore sharp 'shadows' are formed, without which, of course, radiography by means of X-rays (or gamma-rays, which are used for industrial purposes) would be impossible.

In the following sections two important results of the straight line propagation of X- radiation are discussed.

The Inverse Square Law†

Suppose there is a very small source of X-rays at *S* (Fig. 110) and that, at a certain distance from it, there is a screen (opaque to X-rays) having in it a square hole. Suppose also that, on the side of the screen opposite to the source, there is a plane surface (parallel to the screen) on which the radiation falls, after passing through the hole. Then on this surface an area *LMPQ* will be irradiated, which will also be *square*.

Let the distance of this surface from the source be *d*. Then, as *d* is varied, the size of the square *LMPQ* will also vary, getting bigger as *d* increases, and *vice versa*. Now it is clear that of the total X-ray energy

---

* When radiation passes by the edge of an object opaque to it, there is always a certain tendency on the part of the radiation to bend round the edge of the object into what is normally the 'shadow', an effect known as 'diffraction'. Thus, strictly speaking, one should make some qualification to the statement that light, X-rays and gamma-rays travel in straight lines. As, however, the effects of diffraction become less and less easy to detect as the wavelength is decreased, and can be observed only with special equipment in the X-ray region, we shall ignore diffraction in our present studies, and base our treatment on the assumption that both X-rays and gamma-rays *are* propagated in a simple, rectilinear fashion. It must be understood however, that X-ray diffraction is a subject of the utmost importance in other branches of radiology.

† This section has been repeated from 'Mathematics for Radiographers', p. 53–56.

emitted by S in each second, a certain definite fraction of it will pass through the hole in the screen, and this fraction will be constant if the position of the screen (relative to the source) remains fixed. Thus, whatever the value of d, the same amount of radiant energy (E, say)

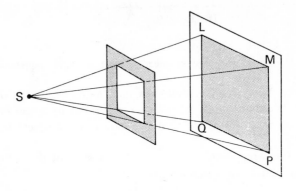

Fig. 110. *LMPQ* is a square area irradiated by S through an aperture of similar shape.

will fall on the area *LMPQ* in each unit of time. When d is small, *LMPQ* will be small, and the energy E will be spread over a relatively small area. The *intensity* of irradiation (which may be defined as the energy which falls in unit time on unit area) will therefore be relatively high. As d is increased, *LMPQ* will increase in size, and in consequence, the same amount of energy E, will be spread over a *larger* area, the intensity of irradiation at the greater distance therefore being less.

Suppose that for two particular positions of the surface on which the radiation is incident, the distances from S are d_1 and d_2 respectively (Fig. 111). Suppose also that l_1 is the length of the side of the (square) area irradiated at distance d_1, and l_2 the corresponding length when the tube distance is d_2. Then the intensity of irradiation at distance d_1 (i.e. the energy in unit time per unit area) is E/l_1^2, and, similarly, the intensity at distance d_2 is E/l_2^2.

$$\therefore \qquad \frac{\text{the intensity at } d_1}{\text{the intensity at } d_2} = \frac{E/l_1^2}{E/l_2^2} = \frac{l_2^2}{l_1^2}.$$

But by similar triangles,

$$\frac{l_2}{l_1} = \frac{d_2}{d_1}.$$

Hence

$$\frac{l_2^2}{l_1^2} = \frac{d_2^2}{d_1^2},$$

and we may write, finally,

$$\frac{\text{intensity at } d_1}{\text{intensity at } d_2} = \frac{d_2^2}{d_1^2},$$

In words we may say:

$$\frac{\text{intensity at first distance}}{\text{intensity at second distance}} = \frac{\text{second distance squared}}{\text{first distance squared}}.$$

This expression is really equivalent to saying that the intensity is *inversely* proportional to the square of the distance,* and hence the result is known as the *Inverse Square Law*.

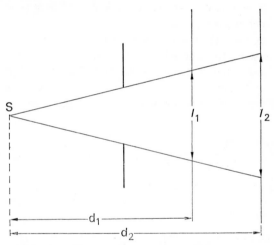

Fig. 111. The length of the side of the irradiated area increases (from l_1 to l_2) with increase of distance (from d_1 to d_2) from the source S.

It must be emphasized that this is a direct geometrical consequence of the rectilinear propagation of the radiation, and that it will apply equally well, for example, to *light*. Implicit in the proof, however, is

* It may actually be written as:

$$\frac{\text{intensity at distance } d_1}{\text{intensity at distance } d_2} = \frac{1/d_1^2}{1/d_2^2} \quad \text{(verify this).}$$

the assumption that the medium through which the radiation travels (on its way to the surface *LMPQ*) is perfectly 'transparent' to the radiation. Thus, in the case of light, a smoky or misty atmosphere in the region between source and screen would cause some of the light to be absorbed and scattered. The energy reaching *LMPQ* would not then be constant, but would depend on the amount absorbed or scattered out of the beam, by the intervening medium. This will obviously complicate the otherwise simple inverse square law relationship between intensity and distance.

In the case of X-rays, the fact that, in general, air will be present as a medium through which the rays must travel has little or no practical effect on the applicability of the Inverse Square Law, except in the case of the less penetrating radiations employed in radiology. Even then, the absorption and scattering caused by the air is not very appreciable unless the X-rays have to travel considerable distances in it—of the order of a metre or so.

To sum up, then, the intensity (i.e. energy in unit time per unit area) will be inversely proportional to the square of the distance from the source, provided that the dimensions of the latter are very small in comparison with the distance involved, and that no appreciable scattering or absorption of the radiation occurs in the medium through which it travels.*

EXAMPLES

1. A surface irradiated by X-rays is at a distance of 40 cm from a small X-ray source. It is moved back 10 cm. If the Inverse Square Law is applicable, express the intensity obtaining in the first position.

   We have $\dfrac{\text{intensity corresponding to distance 50 cm}}{\text{intensity corresponding to distance 40 cm}} = \dfrac{40^2}{50^2} = \dfrac{16}{25}$.

2. The radiation intensity at a distance of 100 cm from a source of X-rays is 50 units. At 60 cm distance, the intensity is found to be 147 units. Can the Inverse Square Law be said to be applicable?

---

* If the source be an extended one, e.g. (in the case of light) a large opalescent electric bulb, then each point on it may be considered as a separate source, and for a surface whose distance from the source is comparable with the dimensions of the latter, the radiation will have come from a large number of different points whose distances from the surface differ appreciably. Obviously the Inverse Square Law will no longer be applicable.

If the Inverse Square Law were applicable:

$$\frac{\text{intensity at 100 cm}}{\text{intensity at 60 cm}} \text{ would equal } \frac{60^2}{100^2},$$

i.e. 36/100, or 0·36.

$$\text{Actually} \qquad \frac{\text{intensity at 100 cm}}{\text{intensity at 60 cm}} = \frac{50}{147} \quad \text{or 0·34.}$$

Thus the Inverse Square Law does not apply in this case, and since the deviation from it is such that the intensity at the greater distance falls below the value which the Inverse Square Law would predict, some absorption and scatter are probably present.

EXERCISES

1. In the case of a certain X-ray unit, it is known that the Inverse Square Law may be considered to hold for distances from the source greater than 50 cm. If the intensity at 70 cm is 50 units, what will the intensity be at (i) 100 cm and (ii) 150 cm?
2. A film is exposed for 4 seconds, at a distance of 100 cm from an X-ray source. What would the exposure have to be at 60 cm in order to produce the same degree of blackening, if the Inverse Square Law is applicable?

THE PINHOLE CAMERA

It is well known that it is possible to form an image on a screen using merely a fine pinhole in an opaque screen (Fig. 112). A very narrow pencil of light from any point, *O*, say, on the object passes through the pinhole to impinge on the screen (at *P*), giving rise there to a small patch of light. The whole image is thus made up of these small patches of light, each of which corresponds to a particular point on the object. As only a very small proportion of the total light emitted from each point on the object is able to pass through the pinhole, the image is a relatively dim one—corresponding to that produced by a lens with a very small aperture indeed. The pinhole must, however, be kept small in order to obtain an image which is sufficiently 'sharp', for increasing the pinhole diameter increases the overlap of the small patches comprising the image, with a resultant blurring effect.

From Fig. 112* it will be seen that the magnification (ratio of size of

* OO′X and PP′X are similar triangles (see 'Mathematics for Radiographers', p. 34).

image to size of object) is given by the ratio of image distance to object distance. Further, it will be realized from the simple geometrical basis of the mode of formation of the image that the latter will be 'in focus' for *any* position of the screen, getting larger (and therefore, of course, less bright) as the distance of the screen from the pinhole is increased.

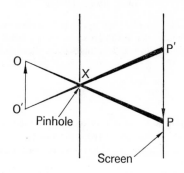

Fig. 112. The principle of the pinhole camera.

Again, the process of image formation does not depend on the wavelength of the light or the angle which the rays make with the axis. In other words the image formed is free from the so-called 'chromatic' and 'spherical' aberration associated with image production by lenses. Provided the pinhole is small enough, the image is reasonably sharp and without distortion, the only objection to such a simple and yet excellent camera being the very small amount of light passed, and consequently the very long exposures necessary unless the object itself is very bright (e.g. the filament of a lamp).

Now X-rays cannot be reflected by mirrors or refracted by lenses in the same way as light. However, the pinhole camera—depending as it does only upon the rectilinear propagation (p. 224) of the radiation for the formation of images—provides a simple and very valuable method of studying the nature and position of the so-called *focal spot* of an X-ray tube, i.e. the area bombarded by the electrons and comprising the source of the X-radiation.

A fine pinhole is made in a lead sheet which is virtually opaque to X-rays. The pinhole is set up on the axis of the X-ray beam at a known distance *d* from the focus (Fig. 113) and an X-ray film is placed a further known distance *D* beyond the pinhole. As described above for light, an image of the focus will then be produced on the film and will become visible on development in the usual way. The dimensions of the actual X-ray source can then be obtained from the image on the film, by

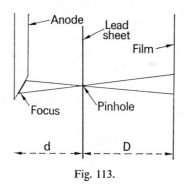

Fig. 113.

multiplying the dimensions of the latter by the ratio of the distance *d* to *D*.

That is, source dimensions = image dimensions $\times \dfrac{d}{D}$.

In most X-ray tubes the focus appears as a replica of the shape of the filament from which the electrons have been accelerated. With a very fine pinhole (say a few thousandths of an inch in diameter) the image obtained is sharp and clear, and even minor damage to the target area can be detected by blurring and distortion of this image.

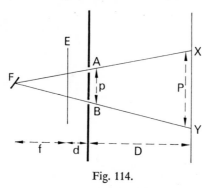

Fig. 114.

Pinhole radiography is also used to check the *position* of the focus, and to determine the focus-skin distance at, say, the end of an applicator.

For this purpose at least *two* pinholes are required (more sometimes being used, but the principle of the method is complete with two). The lead screen, with the pinholes (*A* and *B* in Fig. 114) in it is placed at a known distance *d* from the applicator end, and the film at a distance *D* beyond the pinholes. If the separation of the pinholes is *p*, two images (*X* and *Y*) will be formed on the film with a separation *P* (measured, say, between the centres of the two images). Then the distance *f* of the focus from the applicator end *E* can be determined by a scale drawing (joining the centre of each image to its pinhole and continuing these rays to meet at the focus *F*), or by calculation from the similar triangles *FAB* and *FXY*, whence

$$\frac{AB}{XY} = \frac{\text{ht. of triangle } FAB}{\text{ht. of triangle } FXY},$$

or

$$\frac{p}{P} = \frac{f+d}{f+d+D},$$

from which *f* can be calculated, as *p*, *P*, *d* and *D* are known.

ANSWERS TO NUMERICAL EXERCISES

Chapter 1
page 5
5. 160 cc, 4/5

Chapter 2
page 11
2. 4·4 gm wt, 37°; 3. 39 lb wt, bisecting the angle between them

page 14
1. 28 lb wt, 10 lb wt; 2. 23 lb wt, 19 lb wt

page 17
1. 5 ft; 2. 7 lb; 3. 112·5 lb wt

Chapter 3
page 19
2. $3\frac{1}{2}$ hr; 3. 3 mph

page 22
2. 2·2 ft per sec^2; 3. 10 cm per sec

page 26
1. $20\frac{1}{2}$ mph; 2. $\frac{3}{4}$ mph per sec; 3. 5 mph

page 27
1. 9 ft; 2. 75 ft; 3. 15,750 ft

page 28
1. 2 ft per sec^2; 2. 450 ft; 3. 2 sec

page 29
1. 100 cm per sec; 2. 100 ft; 3. $1\frac{1}{2}$ ft per sec^2

page 30
1. 4·5 sec; 2. 44·1 m per sec; 3. 30·6 m, 24·5 m per sec^2

page 34
1. 0·5 m per sec^2; 2. 0·35 newton; 3. $16\frac{2}{3} \times 10^{-18}$ dyne, 10^4 cm per sec

page 41
2. 3435 joules; 3. 11,600 ergs (approx.); 4. 1470 joules

page 47
2. 1·53 h.p.; 3. 0·065 h.p. (approx.)

Chapter 4

page 56
1. 295·2° A; 2. 63·5° F; 3. 36·9° C

page 61
1. 75 cm of mercury; 2. 73° C

page 64
1. $1\frac{2}{3}$° C

page 68
1. 4200 cal, 1000 joules

Chapter 6

page 119
1. 3·21. 3·2 × 10^{-3} coulombs, 0·02 µF; 2. 0·48 µF, 10 µF; 3. 4 µF, $2\frac{2}{3}$ µF

Chapter 7

page 131
1. 0·62 ohm, 25 cm

page 133
1. 5 ohms; 2. 50 volts, 150 volts, 200 volts; 3. 8 amp

page 135
1. $\frac{1}{4}$ ohms; 2. 49,994 ohms

page 139
1. 250 ohms; 2. 7·24 ohms; 3. $\frac{2}{3}$ amp; 4. 8 ohms

Chapter 8

page 145
1. 1·89 watts; 2. 0·2, 0·4, and 0·6 watts, 14·4 watt-hours; 3. 7·2, 3·6, and 2·4 watts, 158·4 watt-hours; 4. $101\frac{1}{4}$ ohms, 1000 watts; 5. 8·23 min.

Chapter 11

page 145
1. 100 kV; 2. 91 kV, 89% approx.; 3. 0·42 amp

page 195
1. 440 ohms, 7·23 µF; 2. 90 ohms, 0·38 henries, 0·6; 3. 112·5 ohms, 2·99 amp, 0·8

Chapter 12

page 229
1. 24·5 units, 10·9 units; 2. 1·44 sec.

Index